Palliative Care in Critical Care

Editor

TONJA M. HARTJES

CRITICAL CARE NURSING CLINICS OF NORTH AMERICA

www.ccnursing.theclinics.com

Consulting Editor
JAN FOSTER

September 2015 • Volume 27 • Number 3

ELSEVIER

1600 John F. Kennedy Boulevard • Suite 1800 • Philadelphia, Pennsylvania, 19103-2899

http://www.theclinics.com

CRITICAL CARE NURSING CLINICS OF NORTH AMERICA Volume 27, Number 3
September 2015 ISSN 0899-5885, ISBN-13: 978-0-323-39559-5

Editor: Kerry Holland
Developmental Editor: Colleen Viola

Critical Care Nursing Clinics of North America (ISSN 0899-5885) is published quarterly by Elsevier Inc., 360 Park Avenue South, New York, NY 10010-1710. Months of issue are March, June, September, and December. Business and Editorial Offices: 1600 John F. Kennedy Blvd., Suite 1800, Philadelphia, PA 19103-2899. Periodicals postage paid at New York, NY and additional mailing offices. Subscription prices are $150.00 per year for US individuals, $328.00 per year for US institutions, $80.00 per year for US students and residents, $200.00 per year for Canadian individuals, $412.00 per year for Canadian institutions, $230.00 per year for international individuals, $412.00 per year for international institutions and $115.00 per year for Canadian and international students/residents. To receive student/resident rate, orders must be accompanied by name of affiliated institution, data of term, and the *signature* of program/residency coordinator on institution letterhead. Orders will be billed at individual rate until proof of status is received. Foreign air speed delivery is included in all *Clinics* subscription prices. All prices are subject to change without notice. **POSTMASTER:** Send address changes to *Critical Care Nursing Clinics of North America*, Elsevier Health Sciences Division, Subscription Customer Service, 3251 Riverport Lane, Maryland Heights, MO 63043. **Customer Service: 1-800-654-2452 (US and Canada); 314-447-8871 (outside US and Canada). Fax: 314-447-8029. E-mail:** JournalsCustomerService-usa@elsevier.com **(for print support) and** JournalsOnlineSupport-usa@elsevier.com **(for online support).**

Reprints. For copies of 100 or more of articles in this publication, please contact the Commercial Reprints Department, Elsevier Inc., 360 Park Avenue South, New York, New York, 10010-1710; Tel.: 212-633-3874, Fax: 212-633-3820, and E-mail: reprints@elsevier.com.

Critical Care Nursing Clinics of North America is covered in *MEDLINE/PubMed (Index Medicus), International Nursing Index, Nursing Citation Index, Cumulative Index to Nursing and Allied Health Literature,* and *RNdex Top 100.*

Contributors

CONSULTING EDITOR

JAN FOSTER, PhD, APRN, CNS
Formerly, Associate Professor, College of Nursing, Texas Woman's University, Houston; Currently, President, Nursing Inquiry and Intervention Inc., The Woodlands, Texas

EDITOR

TONJA M. HARTJES, DNP, ACNP-BC, FNP-BC, CCRN, CSC
Clinical Associate Professor, Adult Gerontology Acute Care Nurse Practitioner Program, University of Florida, College of Nursing, Gainesville, Florida

AUTHORS

MARIE BAKITAS, DNSc, CRNP, ACHPN, FAAN
Professor, Marie L. O'Koren Endowed Chair, School of Nursing, Associate Director, Center for Palliative and Supportive Care, Division of Geriatrics, Gerontology, and Palliative Care, University of Alabama at Birmingham, Birmingham, Alabama

CHRISTOPHER COLLURA, MD
Assistant Professor of Pediatrics, Division of Neonatal Medicine, Department of Pediatric and Adolescent Medicine, Mayo Clinic College of Medicine, Mayo Clinic, Rochester, Minnesota

PATRICK J. COYNE, MSN, ACHPN, ACNS-BC, FAAN, FPCN
Clinical Director of Palliative Care Services, VCU Medical Center, Richmond, Virginia

J. NICHOLAS DIONNE-ODOM, PhD, RN
Post-doctoral Fellow, School of Nursing, University of Alabama at Birmingham, Birmingham, Alabama

MARIE-CARMELLE ELIE, MD
Associate Professor, Departments of Emergency Medicine, Critical Care, Hospice and Palliative Medicine, University of Florida, Gainesville, Florida

IRENE M. ESTORES, MD
Director, Integrative Medicine Program, Division of General Internal Medicine, University of Florida College of Medicine, Gainesville, Florida

JOYCE FRYE, DO, MBA, MSCE
Chair, Pharmacopeia Revision Committee, Homeopathic Pharmacopeia Convention of the United States, Baltimore, Maryland

TONJA M. HARTJES, DNP, ACNP-BC, FNP-BC, CCRN, CSC
Clinical Associate Professor, Adult Gerontology Acute Care Nurse Practitioner Program, University of Florida, College of Nursing, Gainesville, Florida

JACOBO HINCAPIE-ECHEVERRI, MD
Assistant Professor, Division of Geriatric Medicine, Department of Aging and Geriatric Research, University of Florida College of Medicine, Gainesville, Florida

ARIF KAMAL, MD, MHS
Assistant Professor, Division of Medical Oncology, Duke Palliative Care, Duke Clinical Research Institute, Duke University, Durham, North Carolina

SHERI M. KITTELSON, MD
Assistant Professor and Medical Director, Palliative Care, Division of Hospital Medicine, Department of Medicine, University of Florida, Gainesville, Florida

KEVIN MADDEN, MD
Assistant Professor of Palliative Care, Department of Palliative Care and Rehabilitation Medicine, University of Texas MD Anderson Cancer Center, Houston, Texas

JENNIFER M. MAGUIRE, MD
Assistant Professor, Division of Pulmonary Diseases and Critical Care Medicine, University of North Carolina – Chapel Hill, Chapel Hill, North Carolina

DANIELLE M. NOREIKA, MD, FACP
Medical Director, VCU Inpatient Palliative Services, Assistant Professor of Medicine, Division of Hematology/Oncology and Palliative Care, VCU Medical Center, Richmond, Virginia

LESLYE PENNYPACKER, MD
Clinical Assistant Professor, Medical Director, Palliative Care Program, North Florida/South Georgia Veterans Health System, Malcom Randall VA Medical Center, University of Florida, Gainesville, Florida

CAROLINE M. QUILL, MD, MSHP
Assistant Professor of Medicine, Pulmonary and Critical Care Medicine, Department of Medicine, University of Rochester Medical Center, Rochester, New York

TIMOTHY E. QUILL, MD
Professor of Medicine, Palliative Care Medicine, Department of Medicine, University of Rochester Medical Center, Rochester, New York

LAURENCE M. SOLBERG, MD, AGSF
Ruth S. Jewett Professor, Division of Geriatric Medicine, Department of Aging and Geriatric Research, University of Florida College of Medicine, Gainesville, Florida

BERNARD L. SUSSMAN, MD
Professor of Clinical Medicine, Palliative Care Medicine, Department of Medicine, University of Rochester Medical Center, Rochester, New York

JOANNE WOLFE, MD
Director, Pediatric Palliative Care, Division Chief, Pediatric Palliative Care Service, Department of Psychosocial Oncology and Palliative Care, Children's Hospital Boston, Dana-Farber Cancer Institute, Associate Professor of Pediatrics, Harvard Medical School, Boston, Massachusetts

Contents

> The United States has a changing populace with an increasing number of vulnerable, diverse, and older adults. Of people aged 65 and older, nearly two-thirds suffer from serious comorbidities. Costs associated with chronic illness increase with age and number of conditions. More than 25% of older adults do not have advanced care planning. The current model of health care cannot meet these needs. The initiation of palliative care in the ICU will capture many patients who meet the criteria for palliative care and improve their QOL by management their end-of-life symptoms and reduce unnecessary utilization of health care resources.

> Interdisciplinary teams are at the core of intensive care unit palliative care consultation. They allow health professionals of different disciplines to collaborate in a synergistic fashion to achieve the goals of patients and their families. Interdisciplinary teams can have a variety of members depending on available resources and the goals for its function. There are multiple benefits to highly functioning teams, as well as challenges that may be faced when trying to provide patient care in a team-based setting. Interdisciplinary teams of different structures may provide the ideal support for complex cases in critical care settings.

> Intensive care units provide a wide range of care to patients with serious or life-threatening conditions. This care provides excellent state-of-the-art interventions, often concentrated on meeting national health priorities and performance measures. Overall patient care and the resultant outcomes in the intensive care unit are superb. However, one area that needs improvement is the provision of high-quality palliative care (PC) and end-of-life care. Many providers and administrators now realize implementing PC in the critical care setting is vital to optimal patient outcomes. PC improves patient and family satisfaction and quality of life, reduces length of stay and 30-day readmission rates, and patients can live longer with PC.

> Aggressively managing the symptoms of patients with critical life-limiting illness or terminal disease can improve the quality of life for patients and loved ones, regardless of how much time they have remaining. Palliative symptom management approaches disease in a holistic manner, addressing not only the physical aspect of symptoms but also the psychological, social, and spiritual dimensions of suffering for total symptom relief. Pain is the most common reason for critical care palliative consultation, and using the World Health Organization Pain Ladder to systematically quantify, treat, and titrate pain is effective. Options include both pharmacologic and nonpharmacologic treatment.

> The chronicity of illness that afflicts children in Pediatric Palliative Care and the medical technology that has improved their lifespan and quality of life make prognostication extremely difficult. The uncertainty of prognostication and the available medical technologies make both the neonatal intensive care unit and the pediatric intensive care unit locations where many children will receive Pediatric Palliative Care. Health care providers in the neonatal intensive care unit and pediatric intensive care unit should integrate fundamental Pediatric Palliative Care principles into their everyday practice.

> Patients seek care in the emergency department (ED) for immediate relief of pain or other symptoms. Emergency physicians are trained to provide care that focuses on disease-directed treatment of acute illnesses; the ED is not considered an entry point for palliative care. Despite this, many patients with chronic or end-stage diseases seek treatment in the ED each year. Improving quality of life (QOL) is an overarching principle of palliative care. The ED is poised to improve patients' QOL by providing palliative interventions to manage pain and exacerbations of chronic illnesses or care near the end of life.

> Conventional medicine is excellent at saving lives; however, it has little to offer to address the physical, mental, and emotional distress associated with life-threatening or life-limiting disease. An integrative approach to palliative care in acute care settings can meet this need by creating healing environments that support patients, families, and health care professionals. Mindful use of language enhances the innate healing response, improves communication, and invites patients and families to participate in their care. Staff should be offered access to skills training to cultivate compassion and mindful practice to enhance both patient and self-care.

Over the course of the last half-century, intensive care units have been the setting for many ethical and legal debates in medicine. This article outlines three important domains that lie at the intersection of critical care, palliative care, ethics, and the law: withholding and withdrawal of potentially life-sustaining therapies, making decisions for critically ill patients who lack decision-making capacity, and approaching cases of perceived futility when patients and families still request everything that is medically possible. Important principles and precedents that underlie our understanding of how nurses should approach critically ill patients are reviewed.

Defining the quality of intensive care unit (ICU) care when patients are dying is challenging. Palliative care has been recommended to improve outcomes of dying ICU patients; however, traditional ICU quality indicators do not always align with palliative care. Evidence suggests that some aspects of ICU care improve when palliative care is integrated; however, consensus is lacking concerning the outcomes that should be measured. Overcoming challenges to measuring palliative care will require consensus development and rigorous research on the best way to evaluate ICU palliative care services.

CRITICAL CARE NURSING
CLINICS OF NORTH AMERICA

THE CLINICS ARE AVAILABLE ONLINE!
Access your subscription at:
www.theclinics.com

Preface

Critical Care: Making the Difference with Palliative Care

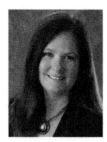

Tonja M. Hartjes, DNP, ACNP-BC, FNP-BC, CCRN, CSC
Editor

Despite our best efforts and extensive use of medical resources, seven out of ten patients with chronic illnesses will die of their disease.[1] Actually, 20% of deaths in the United States are associated with an intensive care unit (ICU) stay, and nearly half of US patients who die in hospitals experience an ICU stay during the last 3 days of life.[2,3] In reality, death is not uncommon in the ICU or emergency department (ED) settings; however, predicting which of our patients will die is often problematic.[4] The implementation of palliative care (PC) in the critical care setting has many benefits and will reduce the burden of disease, so that adequate pain control, symptom management, and social and psychological support may be provided to patients and their families.

This issue of *Critical Care Nursing Clinics of North America* focuses on providing support to implement PC in the critical care setting. The authors provide a wide range of articles devoted to various aspects of PC, thus providing the knowledge to skillfully design, implement, and evaluate a PC program. We begin our issue with the article entitled, "Making the Case for Palliative Care in Critical Care," which describes the evolution of PC over the past several decades. This article provides a framework to discuss PC and its impact on patient care as it is seen today. Other articles range from topics such as creating an interdisciplinary team, determining which patients will benefit from PC, symptom management, to topics such as the evaluation of outcomes criteria. In addition, other topics, such as PC in pediatrics, the ED, integrative medicine, and ethics and law, are included. It is my intention to provide the reader with a comprehensive overview of PC topics, so the reader will then be able to provide evidenced-based practices to improve the outcomes and satisfaction for patients suffering from life-limiting illnesses and for their families.

Crit Care Nurs Clin N Am 27 (2015) ix–x
http://dx.doi.org/10.1016/j.cnc.2015.05.009
0899-5885/15/$ – see front matter © 2015 Published by Elsevier Inc.

ccnursing.theclinics.com

Tonja M. Hartjes, DNP, ACNP-BC, FNP-BC, CCRN, CSC
University of Florida, College of Nursing
Adult Gerontology Acute Care
Nurse Practitioner Program
2900 Southwest 2nd Court
Gainesville, FL 32601, USA

E-mail address:
hartjtm@ufl.edu

REFERENCES

1. Institute for Clinical Systems Improvement. A business case for providing palliative care services across the continuum of care. 2012. Available at: https://www.icsi.org/_asset/40231v/Case-for-Palliative-CareV2.1.pdf. Accessed April 3, 2015.
2. Aslakson RA, Bridges JF. Assessing the impact of palliative care in the intensive care unit through the lens of patient-centered outcomes research. Curr Opin Crit Care 2013;19(5):504–10.
3. O'Mahony S, McHenry J, Blank AE, et al. Preliminary report of the integration of a palliative care team into an intensive care unit. Palliat Med 2010;24(2):154–65.
4. Mirel M, Hartjes T. Bringing palliative care to the surgical intensive care unit. Crit Care Nurse 2013;33(1):71–4.

Making the Case for Palliative Care in Critical Care

Tonja M. Hartjes, DNP, ACNP-BC, FNP-BC, CCRN, CSC

KEYWORDS

- Palliative care • Outcomes • ICU • ED • Communication
- Interdisciplinary teams • Quality of life

KEY POINTS

- Death is pervasive, it affects all people, transcending all races, ethnicities, and socioeconomic and age groups.
- Palliative care should be initiated with the onset of disease and be incorporated with curative care.
- Patients with persistent, progressive, or reoccurring medical conditions should be considered for palliative care interventions.
- The last few months of life are noted to have frequent hospital and/or an intensive care unit admissions.
- Initiating palliative care upon admission to critical care units may improve quality of life for patients and decrease symptom burden and length of stay.

BACKGROUND

Palliative care arose in the 1960s as a means to meet the needs of dying patients at the end of life and was based on hospice philosophies. It consisted mostly of symptom management and psychological support for patients and their families. Historically, health care providers would administer only curative and restorative care at the onset of disease, and palliative care would only be considered when curative treatments had failed.[1,2] Over the past several decades, palliative care has significantly evolved as a result of our changing population in the United States, health care legislation, and the results of research. Palliative care can now be found in both community- and hospital-based settings. Additionally, it is often implemented at various stages of the illness trajectory.[1,3]

The author has nothing to disclose.
Adult Gerontology Acute Care Nurse Practitioner Program, University of Florida, College of Nursing, 1225 Center Drive, PO Box 100187, Gainesville, FL 32610-0187, USA
E-mail address: hartjtm@ufl.edu

In 1990, the World Health Organization defined palliative care as "an approach to care which improves quality of life (QOL) of patients and their families facing life-threatening illness through prevention, assessment, and treatment of pain and other physical, psychological, and spiritual problems."[2] More recently, palliative care is recognized as an adjunct in curative care, becoming a standard of care for patients who have advanced and serious illnesses, such as cancer or heart failure.[1,4] In fact, many organizations such as the American Thoracic Society and the American Society of Clinical Oncology, recommend the integration of palliative care with curative treatments to relieve suffering throughout the course of illness.[1,4] Because of these recommendations, the traditional dichotomous model of palliative care has changed, and palliative care can now be incorporated with curative care early in the course of illness.

Lanken and colleagues[1] further recommend a model of care (**Fig. 1**) that denotes the initiation of palliative care at the time of intensive care unit (ICU) or critical care admission. This model reflects high levels of concurrent curative treatment and palliative care that is individualized for the patient. The figure delineates how curative therapies end just before death, and how palliative care strategies peak around time of death and continue afterward to meet family bereavement needs.

Administrators and providers now understand the significant impact palliative care can have on patient and family outcomes. Anticipated outcomes include:

1. Improved QOL;
2. Improved symptom management;
3. Improved mood;
4. Improved satisfaction (patients, families, and providers);
5. Improved survival;
6. Increase in advanced care planning;
7. Improved health care resource utilization;
8. Improved patient and family support;
9. Decreased hospital readmission rates; and
10. Decreased costs of care.[5]

Providers must reflect on the many benefits of palliative care when considering the timing and setting of initiation.

WHO WILL BENEFIT FROM PALLIATIVE CARE?

The National Consensus Project updated the Clinical Practice Guidelines for Palliative Care in 2013.[3] This edition identified populations that would benefit from palliative

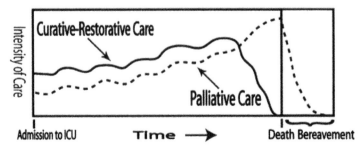

Fig. 1. Palliative care continuum. (*From* Lanken P, Terry P, DeLisser H, et al. Palliative care for patients with respiratory diseases and critical illnesses. Am J Respir Crit Care Med 2008;177:914; with permission of the American Thoracic Society.)

care, and expanded them to include all ages throughout the lifespan. Further recommendations included the addition of all persons living with persistent, progressive, or reoccurring medical conditions. This includes patients who require long-term supportive care as well as patients with developmental or intellectual disabilities or life-limiting illnesses. Moreover, vulnerable and underserved populations were mentioned as a special population (eg, homeless, migrant workers, veterans, prisoners, older adults, and persons with mental illness).[3]

Palliative care can be implemented within most settings in the hospital and across all age groups. Indeed, the number of hospitals with palliative care programs has increased by 157% over the past decade.[6] Despite the expanded definition of who should be included when considering palliative care and the number of growing programs, critical care settings have been slow to implement palliative care across the United States.[7] This is owing in part to the curative and aggressive nature of care within the ICU and emergency departments, which receive approximately 130 million visits per year.[8] Of those admitted to the ICU, more than one-quarter of a million did not survive to discharge.[9] These data indicate that palliative care may benefit a large number of patients in ICU and emergency departments, and should be standard in a hospital setting.

THE CHANGING US POPULATION
Growing Diversity in America

Currently, many large cities within the United States have a large number of minority populations[10] with different cultures and languages. Members of these populations have specific customs, traditions, and expectations and rituals regarding health care and death. In addition, they may have differing levels of health care literacy, which may place them at risk for poor health outcomes. All of these factors potentially create health care disparities and places these patients at greater risk for poor quality, high-cost care near the end of life.[10] Consequently, these patients may benefit from palliative care, which is person centered and adaptable to different languages and cultures. The palliative care team can provide additional layers of assessment, communication, care, and support. Indeed, through an awareness of the patient and families perspective, the palliative care team can facilitate decisions regarding care, improve symptom management, and provide culturally sensitive social support from diagnosis until the time of death.

An Aging Population

By 2030, more than 20% of the US population will be age 65 years or older.[11,12] Additionally, the number of 65-year-old persons who reach the age of 85 years has increased 48 times, compared with more than a century ago.[13] This increase in life expectancy comes with an increased cost. Nearly 80% of adults 65 years and older have 1 or more medical conditions, and this figure increases with age.[14] Heron stated that of the top 10 leading causes of death, heart disease and cancer account for almost one-half of all deaths.[15] Furthermore, the incidence of cancer is expected to increase by 45% between 2010 and 2030.[10]

Additional comorbidities to consider that have an impact on our aging society is Alzheimer's disease and other dementias. Americans who suffer from dementia are expected to grow from 5.5 million people in 2010 to 8.7 million in 2030. The annual costs in 2010 related to the care of persons with dementia were $157 to $215 million dollars.[16] These figures include indirect costs, such as care by family members, and medical and nursing care in the last year of life. The high costs associated with declining health, loss of functional abilities, and the need for institutional care that can occur with age is expected to double by 2050 to 27 million Americans.[10] Overall, 90 million Americans are currently living with a chronic condition. Despite our best efforts, and extensive use of medical resources, 7 out of 10 of these patients with chronic illnesses will die from their disease.[11]

Implementation of palliative care at the onset of disease, when so many Americans currently are living with advanced and serious illnesses, and even more are expected to impact the United States, is a first step to addressing the concern. Palliative care will reduce the burden of disease and ensure that adequate pain control, symptom management, and social and psychological support will be provided to patients and their families.[7,10] Additionally, advanced care planning would be provided, which will impact soaring health care costs and overuse of resources. More support will be provided to the patient and family, such that admissions to the emergency department or readmission rates will decrease, because the patient's symptoms can be managed at home. Finally, when the time arrives, referrals to hospice will be completed, and patients can die at home or at a staffed hospice center instead of in the ICU.

Dying in America

Death is inevitable and transcends all races, ethnicities, and socioeconomic and age groups. In 2011, 2.5 million Americans died according to the Centers for Disease Control and Prevention.[17] Many studies have indicated that, at the time of death, most patients desire to be in control of their care and to die at home with loved ones.[10] Despite this, dying in America has been replaced with an institution-based death, with frequent hospital and ICU admissions within the last months of life.[10] Unfortunately, many of these patients who wish to make decisions regarding their care may not be cognitively or physically able to when death approaches.[10] Regrettably, more than 25% of all older adults over the age of 75 do not have advanced care planning in place.[10] Palliative care, as stated, would safeguard that patients are in control of their care at the end of life through advanced care planning. Health care would be delivered that matches the predetermined patient and family goals of care, thus eliminating frequent trips to the hospital through provision of good symptom management and family support, thus ensuring a better QOL at end of life for the patient.

CLOSING THE GAP: PROVIDING HIGH-QUALITY PALLIATIVE CARE

The Agency for Healthcare Research and Quality published a series of gap analyses to improve quality of patient care. One report focused on *Improving Health Care and Palliative Care for Advanced and Serious Illness* in 2012.[18] Within the *Summary Report*,[19] core components of quality end-of-life care are described. Through these components, outlined in **Box 1**, outcomes related to pain, distress, patient and family satisfaction, communication, advanced care planning, and health care utilization can improve significantly. The Agency for Healthcare Research and Quality goes on to suggest that, to truly improve quality of care, seamless continuity and coordination of care across multiple health care settings and providers is needed. Furthermore, expanding palliative care initiatives past cancer care to other advanced and serious illnesses is also required to improve patient QOL and health care utilization. They also encouraged bridging the gaps in palliative care by addressing broader populations within palliative care, such as pediatrics, diverse cultures, and other health care concerns.

Box 1
Proposed core components for quality end-of-life care

Frequent assessment of physical, emotional, social, and spiritual well-being

Identification and management of emotional distress

Availability of expert-level palliative care in complex situations

Referral to hospice for prognosis of 6 months or less

Access to coordinated care services 24 hours a day

Management of pain and other symptoms

Patient and family counseling

Family caregiver support

Consideration of social needs

Consideration of religious and spiritual needs

Consistent assessment and revision of care plan and goals of care

---

SUMMARY

The United States has a changing populace with an increasing number of vulnerable, diverse, and older adults. Of people aged 65 and older, nearly two-thirds suffer from serious comorbidities.[10] Overall, 90 million Americans suffer with chronic illnesses and despite often aggressive treatment, upwards of 70% of these patients will die from their condition.[11] Progressive and life-limiting illness such as dementia and cancer are also expected to increase by 45% by 2030.[10] Additionally, the costs associated with chronic illness increases with age and the number of chronic conditions. In 2012, the average expenditure for 0 to 1 conditions was $2025 and increased sharply with 6 or more conditions to $32,658.[20]

Unfortunately, more than 25% of older adults do not have advanced care planning, despite having serious chronic conditions.[10] Studies suggest many of these people will frequent the ED, and have hospital and ICU admissions within the last few months of life.[21,22] The current model of health care in the United States is unable to meet the needs of our population of older adults with progressive or serious illnesses and the increasing vulnerable populations.[4] The initiation of palliative care in the ICU will capture many patients who meet the criteria for palliative care and improve their QOL by management their end-of-life symptoms and reduce unnecessary utilization of health care resources.

REFERENCES

1. Lanken P, Terry P, DeLisser H, et al. Palliative care for patients with respiratory diseases and critical illnesses. Am J Respir Crit Care Med 2008;177:912–27.
2. World Health Organization. Cancer pain relief and palliative care: report of a WHO expert committee. Geneva (Switzerland): World Health Organization; 1990. Technical Report Series No. 804. World Health Organization (WHO). 2004. WHO definition of palliative care. Available at: http://www.who.int/cancer/palliative/definition/en. Accessed February 20, 2015.
3. Dahlin C. Clinical practice guidelines for quality palliative care. 3rd edition. National Consensus Project. 2013. Available at: http://www.nationalconsensusproject.org/NCP_Clinical_Practice_Guidelines_3rd_Edition.pdf. Accessed December 3, 2014.

4. Smith T, Temin S, Alesi E, et al. American Society of Clinical Oncology Provisional Clinical Opinion: the integration of palliative care into standard oncology care. J Clin Oncol 2012;30:880–7.
5. Aziz N, Miller J, Curtis JR. Palliative and end-of-life care research: embracing new opportunities. Nurs Outlook 2012;60:384–90.
6. Morrison RS, Meier DE. The National Palliative Care Research Center and the Center to Advance Palliative Care: a partnership to improve care for persons with serious illness and their families. J Pediatr Hematol Oncol 2011;33(suppl 2):S126–31.
7. Nelson JE, Bassett R, Boss RD, et al. Models for structuring a clinical initiative to enhance palliative care in the intensive care unit: a report from the IPAL-ICU Project (Improving Palliative Care in the ICU). Crit Care Med 2010;38(9):1765–72.
8. Centers for Disease Control and Prevention. FastStats – emergency department visits. 2014. Available at: http://www.cdc.gov/nchs/fastats/emergency-department.htm. Accessed January 5, 2015.
9. Society of Critical Care Medicine (SCCM). Critical care units: a descriptive analysis. 2nd edition. Des Plaines (IL): Society of Critical Care Medicine; 2010.
10. IOM (Institute of Medicine). Dying in America: improving quality and honoring individual preferences near the end of life. Washington, DC: The National Academies Press; 2015.
11. Institute for Clinical Systems Improvement. A business case for providing palliative care services across the continuum of care. 2012. Available at: https://www.icsi.org/_asset/40231v/Case-for-Palliative-CareV2.1.pdf. Accessed January 21, 2015.
12. Centers for Disease Control and Prevention. Helping people to live long and productive lives and enjoy a good quality of life. 2011. Available at: http://www.cdc.gov/chronicdisease/resources/publications/aag/aging.htm. Accessed December 2, 2014.
13. AoA (Administration on Aging). A profile of older Americans: 2012. 2012. Available at: http://www.aoa.gov/AoAroot/Aging_Statistics/Profile/index.aspx. Accessed February 4, 2015.
14. Centers for Disease Control and Prevention & the Merck Company Foundation. The state of aging and health in America 2007: executive summary. Whitehouse Station (NJ): The Merck Foundation; 2007.
15. Heron M. Deaths: leading causes for 2010. Natl Vital Stat Rep 2013;62(6):1–97. Available at: http://www.cdc.gov/nchs/data/nvsr/nvsr62/nvsr62_06.pdf. Accessed February 5, 2015.
16. HHS (U.S. Department of Health and Human Services). National plan to address Alzheimer's disease—2013 update. 2013. Available at: http://aspe.hhs.gov/daltcp/napa/NatlPlan2013.shtml#intro. Accessed April 12, 2015.
17. Hoyert DL, Xu J. Deaths: preliminary data for 2011. Natl Vital Stat Rep 2012;61(6):1–52.
18. Dy SM, Aslakson R, Wilson RF, et al. Improving health care and palliative care for and serious illness. Closing the quality gap: revisiting the state of the science. Evidence report No. 208 (Prepared by Johns Hopkins University Evidence-based Practice Center under Contract No. 290-2007-10061-I.) AHRQ Publication No. 12(13)-E014-EF. Rockville (MD): Agency for Healthcare Research and Quality; 2012. Available at: www.effectivehealthcare.ahrq.gov/reports/final.cfm.
19. McDonald KM, Chang C, Schultz E. Closing the quality gap: revisiting the State of the Science. Summary report (Prepared by Stanford-UCSF Evidence-based Practice Center under Contract No. 290-2007-10062-I.) AHRQ Publication No.

12(13)-E017. Rockville (MD): Agency for Healthcare Research and Quality; 2013. Available at: www.effectivehealthcare.ahrq.gov/reports/final.cfm.
20. CMS (Centers for Medicare & Medicaid Services). Chronic conditions among Medicare beneficiaries. Baltimore, MD: CMS; 2012.
21. Aslakson RA, Bridges JF. Assessing the impact of palliative care in the intensive care unit through the lens of patient-centered outcomes research. Curr Opin Crit Care 2013;19(5):504–10.
22. O'Mahony S, McHenry J, Blank AE, et al. Preliminary report of the integration of a palliative care team into an intensive care unit. Palliat Med 2010;24(2):154–65.

Implementing Palliative Care Interdisciplinary Teams: Consultative Versus Integrative Models

Danielle M. Noreika, MD[a],*, Patrick J. Coyne, MSN, ACHPN, ACNS-BC[b]

KEYWORDS

- Interdisciplinary team • Intensive care unit • Palliative care • Team meetings
- Integrative model • Consultative model

KEY POINTS

- Interdisciplinary teams (IDTs) are the core of palliative care consultation.
- IDTs may include providers, nurses, social workers, chaplains, psychologists, physical or occupational therapists, and other allied professionals, based on available resources.
- Highly functioning IDTs have mutual respect, collaborative vision, and shared leadership, and allow constructive dissent.
- Pitfalls experienced by IDTs include time requirements, imbalance of agreement and dissent, lack of resources, and difficulty establishing leadership.
- Palliative consultation in the intensive care unit may occur in an integrative or collaborative fashion.

Mr X is a 60-year-old gentleman with history significant for cardiomyopathy with an ejection fraction of 10% to 15%. He was admitted to the intensive care unit (ICU) secondary to a heart failure exacerbation. He was intubated and placed on a ventilator in the emergency department for respiratory failure. His wife and 2 daughters had never spoken with the patient regarding his wishes in this instance. Mr X was successfully weaned from the ventilator 5 days after admission with aggressive diuresis and rhythm control; however, his overall status remained tenuous. Several hours after extubation his pulmonary status again worsened and after declining reintubation he was placed on bilevel positive airway pressure (BIPAP). Palliative care was consulted and subsequently held a meeting with the patient, his wife and 2 daughters, the patient's cardiologist, and the ICU team. The ICU team and the patient's cardiologist discussed in

None of the authors have any relevant relationships to disclose.
[a] VCU Inpatient Palliative Services, Division of Hematology/Oncology and Palliative Care, VCU Medical Center, PO Box 980230, Richmond, VA 23298, USA; [b] Palliative Care Services, VCU Medical Center, PO Box 980230, Richmond, VA 23298, USA
* Corresponding author.
E-mail address: dnoreika@mcvh-vcu.edu

detail the medical challenges to improve his pulmonary status enough to remove him from high levels of respiratory support. The patient's wife and daughters were able to ask many of the questions regarding his ICU course, and were relieved to talk about them with the participation of the patient. After a thorough discussion of his prognosis, the patient did not want to continue life-prolonging therapies but feared that he would die in significant distress. The palliative physician discussed the tenets of comfort care in this situation and how medications would be used for symptom management rather than life-supportive measures. The implantable cardioverter defibrillator that was still active was reviewed and, consistent with the patient's now clarified goals of care, deactivated by request. After the family meeting, the palliative social worker and chaplain came to meet with the family and provide support that was especially appreciated by the daughters. Through the use of medications, the patient was successfully weaned from BIPAP to high-flow oxygen and was transferred to the palliative care service for ongoing symptom management. He survived for 2 days surrounded by family and with the support of the palliative interdisciplinary team. His family was extremely grateful for the care he received and the integrated support provided by his primary physician, the ICU, and palliative care teams.

INTRODUCTION TO INTERDISCIPLINARY TEAMS

An IDT uses synergistic and interdependent communication from people of multiple disciplines to achieve a common goal.[1] There are multiple other terms that may be applied to this collaborative group, including multidisciplinary, interprofessional, and multiprofessional, depending on the composition of the team. IDTs are present in multiple arenas in health care, including hospital quality improvement, tumor boards, and specialized medical services such as palliative care.[2–5]

Interdisciplinary teamwork is crucial within palliative care. This term is often included in the definition and it is noted to be one of the core elements by the National Consensus Project for Palliative Care. Palliative care patients have complex circumstances with physical, emotional, spiritual, and social needs, as seen with Mr X. Given the multifactorial nature of these cases, a single provider cannot address the physical and medical decision-making aspects of care for the patient and family.[1]

Even in consideration of addressing physical complaints, there are instances in which IDTs are necessary to achieve optimal symptom management in the context of total pain.[6] Multiple benefits of this team approach are found in the literature, including improved symptom control, reduced length of hospital stay, and higher patient and staff satisfaction.[1] When considering Mr X and his family, palliative care was provided by varying physicians (ICU, palliative care, and cardiology), nurses, social workers, volunteers, and chaplains. Any one intervention might have been helpful; however, it was the combination of their actions and interventions that allowed his goals of care to be acted on and improve his satisfaction and quality of life until his death.

FORMATION OF AN INTERDISCIPLINARY TEAM

Given the importance of the IDT to the provision of quality care, knowledge regarding the formation and characteristics of highly functioning teams, and their potential successes and pitfalls within the practice of palliative medicine, is essential. The success of any palliative care service greatly depends on its core team. Multiple members of the palliative IDT collectively contribute to reaching the goals identified by the patient and family. Palliative care teams may include a provider, nurse, social worker, and chaplain. However, professionals from other disciplines such as pharmacy, physical or occupational therapy, psychology, nutrition, and music therapy, as well as volunteers, may be considered, (**Table 1**).[7]

Resources available within the facility or unit are an important consideration when assembling an IDT.[2] Team members will vary, depending on the patient population. For example, the American Academy of Pediatrics recommends pediatric palliative care teams include physicians, nurses, social workers, case managers, spiritual care providers, bereavement specialists, and child life specialists.[5] Furthermore, team members may vary by region. For instance, in Japan the government recommends that palliative care services include a palliative care physician, psychiatrist, nurse, and pharmacist.[8] Although the presence of many disciplines may seem ideal for complex patient situations, there may be a practical limit to how many IDT members to include to facilitate team meetings. Therefore, the World Health Organization recommends teams consisting of 7 or fewer members as the best approach to efficacy.[1]

Medical providers, such as physicians and advanced practice nurses, are frequently found in palliative care IDTs. Providers are responsible for coordinating the physical medical care that the patients receive. At times, a palliative care physician may have direct responsibility for the care of the patient (ie, as the attending on a palliative care unit or service) or may be consulting with the primary medical team. Palliative medical care often consists of management of symptoms (eg, pain, dyspnea, anxiety) as well as helping patients and families to establish goals of care, as was the primary focus for Mr X. Providers may address psychosocial or spiritual concerns for patients but, in general, most care is provided by those with more expertise in these areas within the IDT.[9] Physicians, especially, may need to adjust to working within the construct of an IDT as they may not have been exposed to this structure during their training.[7]

Nurses are a vital component of the palliative care IDT. In hospitals with a palliative care unit, nurses provide the most direct care for the patients as well as are likely to be the ones who spend the most time with patients and families. They often assume the role of advocate for patients especially in regards to symptom management or necessary patient or family support.[10] Palliative nurses must be skilled in the assessment of symptoms related to life limiting illnesses, such as pain, as well as how to communicate these findings to providers. Likewise, psychosocial or spiritual distress can be screened and reported to members of the IDT to be further addressed.[11] Given the time nurses spend with patients and families, they often serve as leaders during the

Table 1 Potential members of palliative care interdisciplinary teams	
Commonly Included	**Included When Available**
Medical provider (physician or advanced practice nurse)	Physical therapist
Nurse	Occupational therapist
Social worker	Psychologist
Chaplain	Dietician
Child life specialist (pediatrics)	Wound care specialist
Volunteer	Pharmacist
	Music therapists
	Art therapist

Data from Walsh D, Caraceni A, Fainsinger R, et al. Palliative medicine. Philadelphia: Saunders Elsevier; 2009.

IDT meetings. They will update other team members on the various dimensions of suffering patients may face. Nurses may also reinforce the medical plan to patients and families.[11] Skilled palliative nurses, when available, play a pivotal role in the care of patients with life limiting illnesses.

Social workers support the psychosocial assessment and management of the palliative patient. Frequently patients report stressors related to insurance, disability, unemployment, or other financial issues. In addition their caregivers may experience distress caused by the financial or social toll of their service or frustration due to their attempts to attain the care that their family member needs.[12] Although social workers are primarily responsible for evaluating the psychosocial concerns of patients and families and helping to devise strategies to address them, experienced palliative social workers can also provide support to other areas of the patient's care. They may provide supportive counseling, assist with goals of care discussions, or reinforce the medical plan from the providers by arranging resources to make it more feasible for the patient and family.[12] For Mr X, the support of a skilled palliative social worker made a significant difference for his daughters in accepting the information discussed by the providers.

Chaplains are the members of palliative IDT's that provide spiritual assessment and support. Many patients find support in their spirituality, which may not be specifically related to a particular religious background, when faced with a life limiting illness. For that reason it is crucial that an open atmosphere to discussion of spirituality be maintained by all members of the IDT. Multiple members of the IDT may be able to screen for issues related to spirituality, in which the chaplain functions to provide in-depth assessment and support. Although the chaplain may be from a specific religious background, their work is usually based in either a nondenominational context or the context of the religion in which the patient participates. Members of the clergy may also work with patients on spiritual matters as ordained representatives of religious denominations. Although members of the clergy may be available in health care systems on request of patients or chaplains who have evaluated the patient, their involvement should not allow for any degree of proselytizing.[13] Spiritual assessment and support is a crucial piece of the care provided by IDT chaplains.

Palliative care IDTs may be supported by other members depending on location and available resources. Physical therapists may work with the team to help improve or maintain functional ability as well as have an adjunctive role to other symptom management efforts.[14] Occupational therapists can offer benefit as well, even to patients near end of life, in helping to tailor movement strategies to their energy level as well as teaching caregivers how to help their loved one achieve their activity goals.[15] Psychologists and psychiatrists if available may be able to provide great benefit to patients via therapeutic interventions (relaxation training, stress management) or medication management of comorbid mental health disorders.[13] Volunteers in hospice and palliative settings have shown increases in family satisfaction with their participation in patient care.[16] Pharmacists, nutritionists, wound care specialists, music and art therapists if available for directed support may be of benefit to the palliative care team as they manage complex patient situations.[13] For pediatric patients child life specialists may assist in providing age appropriate activities to help promote coping with significant illness.[14] IDTs are supported by several professionals whose synergistic care plans serve to improve the care of the palliative patient. The formation of a highly functioning and effective palliative IDT, albeit crucial to provision of high-quality care to patients with life limiting illness, can be challenging.

CHARACTERISTICS OF HIGHLY FUNCTIONING INTERDISCIPLINARY TEAMS

There are many qualities that successful IDTs possess in relation to several themes, including, structure communication, leadership, and so forth.[2] For many of these areas, there is a delicate balance that must be struck to achieve high levels of efficiency. Consideration for the number of varying team members who may be present from different spheres of health care may be remarkably difficult. As teams begin to form, the early stages will require a more open dialogue, self-reflection, and trials to establish the optimal forum for providing patient care. Dysfunctional team dynamics, if left unresolved, can potentially have a negative impact on patient care.[17] Palliative care providers need to be aware of the components of highly functioning teams, as well as team dysfunction, in order to provide optimal care for patients.

One characteristic of a highly functioning IDT relates to structure. As noted above, there are several professionals who may be included within the palliative team, and inclusion of individuals should always be balanced with the goals the team is trying to reach. Individuals who are knowledgeable in palliative medicine and their background fields (eg, occupational therapy, social work) should be sought after.[17] It may be difficult to establish times when all parties are available but to achieve success the IDT has to be dedicated to setting aside ample time to be able meet and thoroughly discuss patient care.[2] In addition to structured meeting times there also needs to be a communication network to be able to access interdisciplinary input for patient care needs that arise in-between sessions. Team members may also establish more in depth discussions, such as case conferences, as a way of learning from challenging patient encounters and further strengthening the group bond.[2]

Even though structure is an important consideration in the formation of an efficient IDT, communication is at the core of the successful palliative care team. The foundation of the team is shared goals for outcomes (which are typically related to improved patient care) among all team members despite each professional being from a different background.[1] The environment needs to support open communication to encourage all team members to contribute to the discussion.[2] Within the IDT to allow for exchange of ideas it is important to foster participation of multiple team members rather than having 1 or 2 people who dominate the conversation.[17]

Well-balanced dissent is a marker of highly effective teams and can be a difficult balance to strike. In order to fully explore team and patient care issues, all team members must feel comfortable not only voicing contrasting ideas but also accepting potential criticisms of their own ideas. Trust, self-confidence, and mutual respect then are key elements of a productive palliative IDT. The ability to provide feedback to each other is also critical to the IDT relationship; if it is sensitive it should be discussed in private so as not to potentially disrupt the individual's reputation within the group.[17] Although each member of the team functions autonomously as a representative of their knowledge and background, having an identifiable leader can assist in providing clear direction to the team and help to ground discussion in team goals.[2] There are several qualities related to communication and structure that are possessed by good IDTs; when they are not present dysfunctional attributes may detract from the efficiency of the team.

PITFALLS OF INTERDISCIPLINARY TEAMS

IDTs can serve to improve clinical outcomes and improve satisfaction of staff and patients, but in the case of team dysfunction, can potentially produce negative patient outcomes.[1,9] There are many potential pitfalls that may commonly produce obstacles within the group and between group members. Newly assembled and well established IDTs will require time to work through these issues successfully.[3]

A commonly cited barrier within an IDT is lack of clear role definition. Although the group dynamic allows for some degree of role variation for members, respect should be given to the experience level of the individual members to foster the trust and collegiality that is necessary for team function.[1] Some degree of conflict and dissent are common and even necessary to achieve optimal group outcomes, however significant imbalances may negatively impact the overall outcome of the IDT and also the dynamic of the team members. Dissention that negatively affects progress may be related to a lack of role clarity or common goals, or incorrect balance of team members and experience levels, which will disrupt the team atmosphere and affect decision making outcomes.[17] Team leaders may serve to navigate the balance of accordance and dissention to allow for sound decisions that are representative of the experience of the group.[17] Unfamiliarity with the interdisciplinary process may also be an obstacle as health care training in multiple fields may not adequately address this tool.[1] Team building exercises and positive reinforcement to individual team members may serve to address this barrier.[17]

In addition to open discussion IDT's must be based on a set of common goals that the group agrees to work toward.[2] As noted above, feedback based on assessment of quality is vital to the IDT; innovation and efficiency may be affected if a team is unable to accept constructive criticism after introspection. Team leaders should consider opportunities that allow for critique and quality improvement such as routine case conferences.[2]

Time management, especially in today's health care setting, is a key pitfall to the functioning of the IDT. Without commitment by all team members to setting aside sufficient time true collaboration and thorough communication will be unlikely to be achieved.[18] Team leaders should encourage efficiency during meetings to maximize time management. Flexible accessibility in between team meetings is necessary to address concerns that require interdisciplinary support and serves to strengthen the team bond.[2] There are multiple barriers to team dynamics that must be overcome in order to achieve a successful palliative care IDT (**Table 2**).

Table 2
Potential interdisciplinary team pitfalls and corrective actions

Potential Pitfall	Potential Corrective Actions
Lack of respect for other team members	Ensure clear role definition Team-building exercises or team training One-on-one feedback for team members Increase positive reinforcement for individual team members
Lack of directed decision making	Ensure correct balance or expertise of team members Clarify common goals Allow open discussion and dissenting opinions
Lack of professional growth	Ensure process for quality improvement Case conferences to discuss selected cases in more depth Open feedback for group processes
Insufficient time	Set aside regularly scheduled time for team meetings Team leader encourages efficiency during meetings Allow informal communication between meetings

Data from Refs.[1,2,5,8,9,11,17,18]

PALLIATIVE CARE CONSULTATION IN THE INTENSIVE CARE UNIT

Most critically ill patients and their families need some degree of palliative care. However, designing a palliative care program that will support the needs of ICU, the staff, and the patient and family is challenging. These challenges may be based on the size of the institution, number of ICU beds, trained clinicians, palliative care awareness among staff, and hospital resources. There are 3 basic models for initiating palliative care within ICUs (**Table 3**): the integrative, the consultative, or, ideally, a model that contains both.[19]

The Integrative Model

In theory, the integrative model speaks to what every provider and nurse should be doing within their ICU practice, which is delivering palliative care at its basic level. The integrative model includes ensuring the requirements of the patient and family are met by assessing their physical, cultural, spiritual, and psychological needs. Basic tenets of the integrative model are improved communication along with pain and symptom management. Communication may be related to present medical issues, interpretation of challenges for return to the patient's baseline, and an understanding of the patient's goals of medical treatment. This model should accomplish basic pain and symptom management of dyspnea, anxiety, or nausea; as well as provide

Table 3
Pros and cons of the main models for integrating palliative care in the ICU

Consultation by Palliative Care Service	Integration by Critical Care Team in Daily ICU Practice
• Expert input from IDT of specialists • Expertise already exists, additional training unnecessary • Empirical evidence of benefit • Continuity of care before, during, and after ICU • Facilitation of transfer out of ICU for end-of-life care, if appropriate	• Availability of palliative care for all ICU patients and families • Palliative care service not required • Clearly acknowledges importance of palliative care as core element of intensive care • Systematization of ICU work processes promotes reliable performance of palliative care
• Requires palliative care service with adequate staffing and other resources • Palliative care clinicians may be seen as outsiders in ICU • Consultants may lack familiarity with biomedical and nursing aspects of critical care • Activities of palliative care and ICU teams may overlap and/or conflict • Consultants must rapidly establish effective relationship with patients and families • Fragmentation of care may be compounded • ICU team may have less incentive to improve palliative care knowledge and skills	• Depends on commitment of critical care clinicians and supportive ICU culture • Requires dedication of staff and other resources that may be lacking in ICU • Requires handoff to new team for post-ICU palliative care for patients who cannot benefit from or no longer need the ICU

From Nelson J, Bassett J, Boss R, et al. Models for structuring a clinical initiative to enhance palliative care in the intensive care unit: a report from the IPAL-ICU Project (Improving Palliative Care in the ICU). Crit Care Med 2010;38(9):1769; with permission.

consults with professionals such as chaplains, social workers, and/or child life specialists. Use of this model requires some basic education and ongoing training, as well as monitoring, to determine benefit and effectiveness. An ongoing assessment of patients within ICUs using triggers to highlight those most at risk for poor outcomes may improve the awareness, impact, and scope of the integrative model.

Triggers are a set of predetermined criteria or conditions that alert the ICU providers of the potential need for palliative care services. Examples include patients who have been hospitalized in the ICU in the previous 3 months, patients older than the age of 75 years with one or more comorbidities, and patients approaching decisions related to life-prolonging treatments such as dialysis, pressor therapy, feeding tubes, or tracheostomies. Essentially, triggers should identify patient populations that may experience poor outcomes. Many other examples exist and can be tailored to meet the needs of the ICU as well as the greater institution. See the article by Hartjes elsewhere in this issue for further exploration of triggers.

The Consultative Model

The consultative model allows for the input of individuals, outside of the ICU, with specialty training in palliative care. Team members may include providers; nurses; chaplains; psychologists; social workers; speech, occupational, and physical therapists; nutritionists; and specially trained volunteers. The palliative care consultative team brings a coordinated approach to palliative care throughout various hospital settings. Team members assist in treating challenging pain, symptom management, communication concerns such as family discord, understanding of unique cultural and spiritual challenges, and provide many more benefits. The utilization of a palliative care service may be for specific consults or as a resource to round daily with the ICU team. Although rarely available around the clock, when present the team offers help and support for the ICU staff with the most challenging patient and family situations or those experiencing life-limiting diseases. Moral distress is frequently a nursing concern in the ICU where there is concern regarding medical futility and patient suffering.[20] Palliative care can offer support for staff in challenging and emotionally draining or morally distressing patient or family-care situations.[21] The palliative care service may also provide continuity of care and decrease anxiety of patients and families as transfer out of the ICU occurs.

SUMMARY

IDTs are the core of palliative medicine practice. The patients cared for by a palliative service often have complex cases and a unique set of needs. Frequently, in addition to physical symptoms that need to be addressed, there are a multitude of other concerns in psychological, social, spiritual, and other areas. Given the diverse needs of these patients, the IDTs offer a variety of professionals who work together to create care plans that address the whole patient (including their family). There are several professions generally found in palliative care IDTs. The providers (physicians and advanced nurse practitioners) are responsible for the care of the physical symptoms as well as guiding goals for therapy. Nurses provide direct care for patients and often are the strongest link of the team with the patient and their families; offering a wealth of assessment information to the team. Social workers assess and help to arrange support for psychosocial issues. Chaplains may assist with psychosocial issues as well as assessment of spiritual matters. Other professionals may be involved with IDTs, including physical therapists, occupational therapists, dieticians, psychologists, wound care specialists, volunteers, music therapists, and so forth.

There are several hallmarks of effective IDTs. Two important themes are structure and communication. Teams must be aware of the multiple pitfalls that may disrupt group outcomes, including lack of time commitment, absence of clearly defined roles, leadership deficiencies, and not identifying a concrete team goal to work toward.

Palliative care IDTs often collaborate with consulting services such as the ICU. IDTs work within the ICU may be on a consultative or integrative basis depending on the needs and team dynamic at each institution. Interdisciplinary care, which allows for synergy of multiple dedicated professionals of different backgrounds, provides the foundation for the positive outcomes made by palliative teams in the lives of patients and families.

REFERENCES

1. Youngwerth J, Twaddle M. Cultures of interdisciplinary teams: how to foster good dynamics. J Palliat Med 2011;14(5):650–4.
2. Nancarrow S, Booth S, Ariss S, et al. Ten principles of good interdisciplinary team work. Hum Resour Health 2013;11:19.
3. Santana C, Curry L, Nembhard I, et al. Behaviors of successful interdisciplinary hospital quality improvement teams. J Hosp Med 2001;6(9):501–6.
4. Fennell M, Das I, Clauser S, et al. The organization of multidisciplinary care teams: modeling internal and external influences on cancer care quality. J Natl Cancer Inst Monogr 2010;2010(40):72–80.
5. Ogelby M, Goldstein R. Interdisciplinary care: using your team. Pediatr Clin North Am 2014;61(4):823–34.
6. DelFabbro E. Assessment and management of chemical coping in patients with cancer. J Clin Oncol 2014;32(16):1734–8.
7. Wiebe L, Von Roenn J. Working with a palliative care team. Cancer J 2010;16(5): 488–92.
8. Nakazawa Y, Kizawa Y, Hasizume T, et al. One year follow up of an educational inter-vention for palliative care consultation teams. Jpn J Clin Oncol 2014;44(2):172–9.
9. O'Connor M, Fisher C. Exploring the dynamics of interdisciplinary palliative care teams in providing psychosocial care: everybody thinks that everybody can do it and they can't. J Palliat Med 2011;14(2):191–6.
10. Dobrina R, Tenze M, Palese A. An overview of hospice and palliative care nursing models and theories. Int J Palliat Nurs 2014;20(2):75–81.
11. Goldsmith J, Ferrell B, Wittenberg-Lyles E, et al. Palliative care communication in oncology nursing. Clin J Oncol Nurs 2013;17(2):163–7.
12. Otis-Green S, Sidhu R, Del Ferraro C, et al. Integrating social work into palliative care for lung cancer patients and families: a multidimensional approach. J Psychosoc Oncol 2014;32(4):431–46.
13. Walsh D, Caraceni A, Fainsinger R, et al. Palliative medicine. Philadelphia: Saun-ders Elsevier; 2009.
14. Chiarelli P, Johnston C, Osmotherly P. Introducing palliative care into entry-level physical therapy education. J Palliat Med 2014;17(2):152–8.
15. Burkhardt A, Ivy M, Kannenberg M, et al. The role of occupational therapy in end of life care. Am J Occup Ther 2011;65(6):S66–75.
16. Candy B, France F, Low J, et al. Does involving volunteers in the provision of palli-ative care make a difference to patient and family wellbeing? A systematic review of quantitative and qualitative evidence. Int J Nurs Stud 2015;52(3):756–68.
17. Blackmore G, Persaud D. Diagnosing and improving functioning in interdisci-plinary health care teams. Health Care Manag 2012;31(3):195–207.

18. Xyrichis A, Lowton K. What fosters or prevents interprofessional teamworking in primary and community care? A literature review. Int J Nurs Stud 2008;45:140–53.

19. Nelson J, Bassett J, Boss R, et al. Models for structuring a clinical initiative to enhance palliative care in the intensive care unit: a report from the IPAL-ICU Project (Improving Palliative Care in the ICU). Crit Care Med 2010;38(9):1765–72.

20. Meltzer LS, Huckabay LM. Critical care nurses' perceptions of futile care and its effect on burnout. Am J Crit Care 2004;13:202–8.

21. Weissman D, Nelson J, Campbell M. Palliative care consultation in the ICU. Available at: https://www.capc.org/fast-facts/253-palliative-care-consultation-icu/. Accessed February 21, 2015.

Predicting Which Patients Will Benefit From Palliative Care: Use of Bundles, Triggers, and Protocols

Tonja M. Hartjes, DNP, ACNP-BC, FNP-BC, CCRN, CSC

KEYWORDS

- Palliative care • Triggers • Protocols • End-of life care • ICU • Bundles
- Communication • Interdisciplinary teams

KEY POINTS

- The provision of high-quality palliative and end-of life care in the ICU is a national health priority.
- The implementation of PC should be consistent and standardized with the use of bundles, triggers, and protocols to ensure continuity of PC among various hospital settings.
- Palliative care in the ICU improves patient outcomes and satisfaction.

INTRODUCTION

Intensive care units (ICUs) provide a wide range of care to patients with serious or life-threatening conditions. This care provides excellent state-of-the-art interventions, often concentrated on meeting national health priorities and performance measures. Overall patient care and the resultant outcomes in the ICU are superb. However, one area that needs improvement is the provision of high-quality palliative and end-of life care.[1]

Approximately 20% of deaths in the United States are associated with an ICU stay, and nearly half of US patients who die in hospitals experience an ICU stay during the last 3 days of life.[2,3] However, because of a lack of palliative care (PC) in critical care units, the Institute of Medicine[4] has published a call to action to implement PC in the ICU and emergency department (ED). The long-term goal is to reduce the burden of disease, provide adequate pain control and symptom management, and administer social and psychological support to patients and their families.[5]

Many providers and administrators now realize implementing PC in the critical care setting is vital to optimal patient outcomes. PC improves patient and family satisfaction and quality of life, it reduces length of stay (LOS) and 30-day readmission rates,

The author has nothing to disclose.
Adult Gerontology Acute Care Nurse Practitioner Program, University of Florida, College of Nursing, 1225 Center Drive, PO Box 100187, Gainesville, FL 32610-0187, USA
E-mail address: hartjtm@ufl.edu

and patients can actually live longer with PC.[6,7] So the question is not "Should we implement PC," but rather "How do we implement PC" and "How do we predict which patients will benefit from PC?"

IMPLEMENTING PALLIATIVE CARE

The Center to Advance Palliative Care 2014 recognized the need for PC in the ICU and ED and created Improving Palliative Care in the ICU and Emergency Department (the IPAL-ICU and IPAL-ED Projects). These resources outline five key steps to consider when implementing a PC program[8–10]: (1) identify all stakeholders, (2) conduct a needs assessment, (3) develop an action plan, (4) evaluate progress, and (5) create a culture of support and change in the unit.

Step 1: Identify All Stakeholders

Hospital and ICU administrative support, which is vital to program success, should be obtained at the start. Next, a multidisciplinary, PC team is assembled. Members should be interdisciplinary, and at a minimum include medical directors, nurse managers, physicians, nurses, chaplains, social workers, pharmacy representatives, and nurse educators.

Step 2: Conduct a Needs Assessment

The PC team needs to ask key questions, such as "Why do we need PC?" Answers to this question help determine unit needs and direct the next steps. Perhaps readmission rates or mortality rates are elevated. Possibly the ICU is having difficulty with daily "bed crunches" and use of health care resources. Conceivably patient satisfaction scores with care or treatment of pain scores are poor. Not only do PC teams ultimately improve performance measures, but they also improve patient and family satisfaction and quality of life. Once the PC team completes the needs assessment, it should define the unit's opportunities for improvement and determine the resources for PC, which may be integrative, consultative, or a combination.[5] Team members may ask questions, such as "Will the facility have a PC consultative team?" "Who will the team members be?" "Will we integrate primary PC aspects into the unit?" Regardless of how the PC team implements PC, it should be done in a way that benefits the highest number of patients, with the available resources.

Step 3: Develop an Action Plan

For this step, the PC team should revisit the needs assessment, identify and prioritize problems, and set timely and achievable goals. Then, the PC team should identify potential resources and develop an action plan. The implementation of PC may vary among facilities and units based on Step 2.

Step 4: Evaluate Progress

The outcomes that are frequently measured are determined from the needs assessment. They can include knowledge and perceptions of PC, consultation appropriateness and volume, LOS, readmission rates, pain scores, mortality and patient and family satisfaction, just to name a few. An entire article in this journal is devoted to outcomes measurement in PC.

Step 5: Create a Culture of Support and Change

The PC team must develop and foster a supportive culture and environment, which are vital for the successful implementation of a PC program. Communication must be open and all key stakeholders must have a voice in program design, implementation, and evaluation.

It is important that PC teams begin program implementation by identifying and collaborating with stakeholders, who can provide key insights to the target patient population. In addition, team members need to identify areas of improvement and conduct needs assessments to create a successful program. Although PC program design and implementation vary by hospital, using a standardized approach facilitates progress.

IMPROVING PATIENT CARE WITH USE OF BUNDLES, TRIGGERS, AND PROTOCOLS

Next an overview of two models of PC will be discussed, along with various strategies that have been implemented within critical care units. These may be helpful in determining next steps in identifying and predicting which patients will benefit most from PC efforts.

INTEGRATIVE STRATEGIES

Lanken and colleagues[11] suggest that PC should begin on admission to the ICU, and be used in conjunction with curative therapies. Staff in the ICU do not need to be certified to provide primary PC interventions. An integrative approach incorporates PC principles into the patient-centered, daily practice of the unit and the providers.[12] Examples include the following:

- Effective and timely communication between patients, their families, and ICU providers.
- Education of patients and families, who are included in decision-making processes.
- Ensuring the alignment of treatment plans with patients' goals.
- Provision of pain relief and appropriate management of symptoms.
- Initiating discussion of social and spiritual support.
- Considerations for transitions of care postdischarge.

Critical care patients condition can change rapidly; with this integrative approach, patient care needs are continually evaluated and acted on. Typically, use of a formal "consultative" PC team is not required unless an unusual situation occurs.

CONSULTATIVE STRATEGIES

The hallmark of the consultative approach is the PC interdisciplinary team. This team is external to the critical care setting, and has special knowledge and experience in PC. Although the implementation of this approach varies the consultative care team assist patients as they transition between units to ensure care continuity.

The scope of the consultation depends on facility and unit preferences. The team can assist with determination of health care surrogates, communication of prognosis, treatment options, goals of care, and advanced directives. The PC team can also be a source of support and guidance to providers. Assisting when there is a lack of agreement among family members about treatment and goals of care. Within this context, the PC team may provide family caregivers with respite from caregiving, spend time with patients and their families, help manage symptoms, and provide spiritual support. A consultative approach ensures continuity of PC with the hospital as patients' transition between units.

PALLIATIVE CARE BUNDLES

PC bundles are a series of independent best practice interventions that can improve quality of care and patient outcomes. Critical care units are familiar with the concept of bundled care. The Institute for Healthcare Improvement has been at the forefront and has identified several bundles of care to prevent hospital-acquired infections and other hospital-acquired events (eg, the ventilator bundle).[13] In 2006, Nelson and colleagues[14] introduced PC bundles within the Veterans Healthcare Administration through the "Transformation of the ICU" program. This program integrated an approach named the Care and Communication Bundle, which used nine PC quality measures to improve communication and care provided to ICU patients:

- Identification of medical decision maker
- Determination of advance directive status
- Investigation of resuscitation preference
- Distribution of family information leaflet
- Regular pain assessment
- Optimal pain management
- Offer of social work support
- Offer of spiritual support
- Interdisciplinary family meeting

Several iterations of these bundles are noted within the literature, but generally, the PC process measures are distributed by LOS. Nelson and colleagues[14] describe the following:

- Day 1: Identify decision maker, complete advanced directives, determine code status, assess and manage reoccurring pain, and provide information leaflets
- Day 3: Visits by the social worker and chaplain
- Day 5: Conduct a meeting between the family and the interdisciplinary PC team

In 2013, Black and coworkers[15] implemented a statewide two-day bundle process (Days 1 and 3) across multiple ICU settings (eg, open vs closed, teaching vs community, medical vs surgical) and demonstrated a profound improvement in primary PC interventions. This Care and Communication Bundle incorporated aspects of care already used in many ICUs, and as a result it can readily be implemented and measured. To ensure sustainability of any program, including its use in policy with documentation templates and including them as performance measures is recommended.

PALLIATIVE CARE TRIGGERS

Weissman and Meier[12] describe the use of "triggers" to identify patients who are in need of PC interventions. Triggers can be objective, patient-, or disease-specific criteria. For example, triggers may be the day of hospitalization; readmission within 30 days; or the diagnosis of serious disease, such as metastatic cancer. There are five steps for the successful development and implementation of triggers within a critical care setting[12]:

1. Identify or define the facilities' unmet goals.
2. Evaluate the PC team's resources. Triggers typically increase PC consultation volumes.
3. Secure buy-in from key stakeholders.

4. Select consultation triggers, which are facility and unit specific. Clinicians must be involved in this process. Trial and error is to be expected and required to evaluate success of triggers.
5. Determine how the triggers will be implemented. This can include an initial internal review to determine need for an external PC consultation, or a direct PC consultation from the trigger.

Additionally, Weissman and Meier[12] describe a two-step approach (with primary and secondary criteria) that may be used to assess for PC consultation or interventions.[12] Primary criteria are broad indicators to screen patients at risk. These can include such items as (1) decline in function or age; (2) complex care requirements, such as mechanical ventilation and tube feedings; (3) difficult to control symptoms; (4) multiple admissions for the same illness over the past year; (5) the "surprise question" ("Would you be surprised if the patient died with the next 12 months or before reaching adulthood?"); (6) ICU admission greater than 7 days; and (8) disagreement with treatment plans and goals.[12]

Secondary criteria are more specific indicators and can include (1) admission from long-term care facility, (2) metastatic disease, (3) out-of-hospital arrest, (4) current hospice patient, (5) elderly or cognitively impaired, (6) awaiting or deemed inappropriate for transplant, and (7) consideration of life-sustaining treatment (eg, dialysis, feeding tube, tracheostomy for long-term ventilation).[12]

Hua and coworkers[1] completed a retrospective cohort study that reviewed ICU admissions across the United States from 2001 to 2008 to determine the prevalence of patients meeting one or more PC triggers. The results revealed 13.8% to 19.7% of all ICU admissions met one or more primary triggers for PC. Additionally, those patients requiring a PC consultation, 85.4% were captured by one of five triggers: (1) ICU admission 10 days or more, (2) multisystem organ failure of at least three systems, (3) stage IV malignancy, (4) status post cardiac arrest, and (5) intracerebral hemorrhage (ICH) requiring mechanical ventilation. The study concluded that one in seven ICU admissions met at least one PC trigger and one in five was noted to meet multiple PC triggers. These results were consistent among regions in the United States and differing types of ICUs. Currently, there are not enough certified PC providers to meet the needs for PC services in the hospital. Implementation of a PC program does not require expertise in PC; however, a basic understanding of the process and skills is necessary.

USE OF GUIDELINES AND PROTOCOLS WITHIN PALLIATIVE CARE

Decision-support tools, such as clinical guidelines and protocols, were developed to aid providers in decision-making and to standardize and ensure the provision of evidenced-based care. The use of PC guidelines and protocols improves overall quality of care, communication between members of the interdisciplinary team, and appropriate use of resources.

Guidelines of care are general overviews of a condition similar to a textbook, and provide information regarding themes of care. However, they provide little instruction about specific decisions of care. An example of a PC guideline is the Clinical Practice Guidelines for Quality Palliative Care 3rd Ed[3] from the National Consensus Project.[16]

Protocols, however, are specific instructions that the provider can use to make clinical decisions. Examples include algorithms, clinical pathways, and order sets. Examples of protocols and order sets that can facilitate and standardize PC include (1) pain management, (2) sedation management, (3) ventilator weaning and termination, and (4) withdrawal of life. Another example includes a rapid two-stage screening protocol implemented in 2011 by Glajchen and colleagues[17] to improve PC referrals of the elderly in the ED. In this study 22% of patients 65 years of age and older who visited the ED met criteria for PC referrals.

ALTERNATIVE APPROACHES FOR PALLIATIVE CARE INTERVENTIONS

Although PC consultations, bundles, and triggers are commonly used strategies to implement PC programs in critical care settings, other approaches, such as varied interventions or as a combination of approaches, can also be used.

The American Association of Critical Care Nurses created the Promoting Excellence in Palliative Care and End-of-Life resource site.[18] Resources and other best practices are available on their Web site. Some of their innovative PC approaches include (1) the No One Dies Alone intervention, in which volunteers sit with dying patients; (2) debriefings for staff after patient death; (3) hospice consultations for bereaved families; (4) cross-cultural awareness and accommodation; (5) "Getting to Know Me" posters, which include personal information and pictures about the patient; and (6) PC grand rounds and morbidity and mortality meetings.

As an example of a combination strategy, in 2013 Huffines and coworkers[19] described implementation of a combination PC bundle and clinical trigger algorithm for determining PC interventions. The traditional Care and Communication Bundle was implemented at Days 1, 3, and 5. In addition, predetermined clinical triggers were assessed each day from the prior timeframe. If any of the clinical triggers had occurred, the next days' events were expedited in anticipation of increased levels of care. Outcomes included an overall improved patient and family satisfaction and observed ICU teamwork.

PC in the ED, which has been slowly developing over the past 5 years, focuses on pain and symptom management and hospice referrals. However, one university medical center in the southeast is considering innovative approaches to implementing PC in the ED: a hospice nurse navigator and PC based on team and admission International Classification of Diseases (ICD)-10 code. The first approach includes placing a Hospice Nurse Navigator in the ED. This navigator provides a single source contact for patients and their families to provide identification of those at risk or in need of PC interventions during a crisis. They act as a liaison between the patient/family and the health care providers in the ED to maintain treatment with patient goals of care. This may include adequate symptom management, continuing outpatient do-not-resuscitate status, de-escalation of ED therapy, prevention of in-hospital admission, or discharge to home with hospice (Kittelson, personal communication, 2015).

The second approach includes implementing a "primary PC" method by identification of PC patients by the ED team on admission by service and admission ICD-9-CM code. This university medical center is a level 1 trauma center, and as such many unexpected traumatic events are seen. Opportunities to intervene with PC interventions have identified a patient cohort with a poor survival rate. They include ICD-9-CM 431.0 (severe ICH) and ICD-9-CM 853.0 (other unspecified hemorrhage) present on admission and trauma alert. A feasibility study was performed before implementing the process, which identified 173 patients from January 1 to August 31, 2014, from a de-identified patient encounter database.[20] Currently the university medical center is exploring the idea of implementing a combined neurosurgical ICU primary PC project and an ED PC program with patients identified with ICH.[20]

SUMMARY

PC should begin on admission to the ICU, in conjunction with curative therapies, because the benefits of PC are well known. They can include decreased health care costs because of reduced hospitalization, ICU LOS, and 30-day readmission rates; improved pain scales and patient and provider satisfaction scores; improved quality of life; and an actual decrease in mortality.[6,7] Despite these benefits, PC within critical care has been slow to advance.

Five key steps are necessary when devising a PC program: (1) identify all stake-holders, (2) conduct a needs assessment, (3) develop an action plan, (4) evaluate progress, and (5) create a culture of support and change in the unit.[8–10] All five steps are crucial in the process, and omission of any one step affects the success of the program. Whether one chooses an integrative or consultative approach when implementing PC, various strategies may be used based on the needs of the facility and/or unit. Additionally, regardless of the process, the use of PC bundles, triggers, guidelines, and protocols assist the identification of patients in need of PC services and standardizes the interventions provided.

REFERENCES

1. Hua MS, Li G, Blinderman CD, et al. Estimates of the need for palliative care consultation across United States intensive care units using a trigger-based model. Am J Respir Crit Care Med 2014;189(4):428–36.
2. Aslakson RA, Bridges JF. Assessing the impact of palliative care in the intensive care unit through the lens of patient-centered outcomes research. Curr Opin Crit Care 2013;19(5):504–10.
3. O'Mahony S, McHenry J, Blank AE, et al. Preliminary report of the integration of a palliative care team into an intensive care unit. Palliat Med 2010;24(2):154–65.
4. Institute of Medicine (IOM). Dying in America: improving quality and honoring individual preferences near the end of life. 2014. Available at: http://www.iom.edu/Reports/2014/Dying-In-America-Improving-Quality-and-Honoring-Individual-Preferences-Near-the-End-of-Life.aspx. Accessed November 13, 2014.
5. Nelson JE, Bassett R, Boss RD, et al. Models for structuring a clinical initiative to enhance palliative care in the intensive care unit: a report from the IPAL-ICU project (Improving Palliative Care in the ICU). Crit Care Med 2010;38(9):1765–72.
6. Ouchi K, Wu M, Medairos R, et al. Initiating palliative care consults for advanced dementia patients in the emergency department. J Palliat Med 2014;17(3): 346–50.
7. Institute for Clinical Systems Improvement. A business case for providing palliative care services across the continuum of care. 2012. Available at: https://www.icsi.org/_asset/40231v/Case-for-Palliative-CareV2.1.pdf. Accessed January 17, 2015.
8. Center to Advance Palliative Care. Improving palliative care in emergency medicine: improvement tools. 2014. Available at: http://www.capc.org/ipal/ipal-em/improvement-and-clinical-tools. Accessed October 21, 2014.
9. Hartjes T, Meece L, Horgas A. Implementing palliative care in the ICU: providing patient and family centered care. Nursing 2014. Crit Care 2014;9(4):17–22.
10. Bryant EN, Quest TE, DeSandre PL, et al. Getting started: organizing an ED palliative care initiative: a technical assistance monograph from the IPAL-EM Project. 2011. Available at: http://ipal.capc.org/downloads/ipal-em-getting-started.pdf. Accessed December 22, 2014.
11. Lanken P, Terry P, DeLisser H, et al. Palliative care for patients with respiratory diseases and critical illnesses. Am J Respir Crit Care Med 2008;177:912–27.
12. Weissman D, Meier D. Identifying patients in need of a palliative care assessment in the hospital setting: a consensus report from the Center to Advance Palliative

Care. J Palliat Med 2011;14(1):1–8. Available at: http://mhcc.dhmh.maryland. gov/Documents/Health_Community/JPM_article.pdf. Accessed October 24, 2014.

13. Institute for Healthcare Improvement (IHI). Evidenced-based care bundles. 2015. Available at: http://www.ihi.org/topics/Bundles/Pages/default.aspx. Accessed October 24, 2014.

14. Nelson JE, Mulkerin CM, Adams LL, et al. Improving comfort and communication in the ICU: a practical tool for palliative care performance measurement and feedback. Qual Saf Health Care 2006;15:264–71.

15. Black M, Vigorito M, Curtis JR, et al. A multifaceted intervention to improve compliance with process measures for ICU clinician communication with ICU patients and families. Crit Care Med 2013;41:2275–83.

16. Dahlin C. Clinical practice guidelines for quality palliative care 3rd Ed 2013 National Consensus Project. Available at: http://www.nationalconsensusproject. org/NCP_Clinical_Practice_Guidelines_3rd_Edition.pdf. Accessed October 19, 2014.

17. Glajchen M, Lawson R, Homel P, et al. A rapid two-stage screening protocol for palliative care in the emergency department: a quality improvement initiative. J Pain Symptom Manage 2011;42(5):657–62.

18. American Association of Critical Care nurses (AACN). Promoting excellence in palliative care and end-of-life resource kit. 2014. Available at: http://www.aacn. org/WD/Palliative/Content/PalAndEOLHome.content?menu=Practice. Accessed January 4, 2015.

19. Huffines M, Hohnson K, Smitz Naranjo L, et al. Improving family satisfaction and participation in decision making in an intensive care unit. Crit Care Nurse 2013; 33(5):56. Available at: http://www.aacn.org/wd/Cetests/media/C1353.pdf. Accessed January 4, 2015.

20. Hill A. Palliative care consultation program in the emergency department: a feasibility study. DNP Capstone Project University of Florida; 2015.

Palliative Care Symptom Management

Sheri M. Kittelson, MD[a],*, Marie-Carmelle Elie, MD[b,c,d], Leslye Pennypacker, MD[e]

KEYWORDS

- Palliative care • Hospice • Symptom management • Pain • Dyspnea

KEY POINTS

- Aggressively managing the symptoms of patients with critical life-limiting illness or terminal disease can improve the quality of life for patients and their loved ones, regardless of how much time they have remaining.
- Palliative symptom management approaches disease in a holistic manner, addressing not only the physical aspect of symptoms but also the psychological, social, and spiritual dimensions of suffering for total symptom relief.
- Pain is the most common reason for critical care palliative consultation, and using the World Health Organization Pain Ladder to systematically quantify, treat, and titrate pain is effective.
- Treatment options include both pharmacologic and nonpharmacologic management.

INTRODUCTION

Palliative care is a relatively new discipline, and over the past 10 years programs have grown rapidly. Since 2000, the number of hospitals with inpatient palliative care teams has increased by nearly 148%, including 66% of all hospitals with more than 50 beds.[1] Experts believe that 5% to 10 % of all hospital admissions qualify for inpatient palliative care consultations, but this number depends on the hospital patient population.[1] Palliative care consultations typically include: symptom management, prognosis, goals of care, advance care planning such as code status/completion of advance directives, and psychosocial and spiritual support.

The authors have nothing to disclose.
[a] Palliative Care, Division of Hospital Medicine, Department of Medicine, University of Florida, PO Box 100238, Gainesville, FL 32610-0238, USA; [b] Department of Emergency Medicine, University of Florida, 1515 Southwest Archer Road, Gainesville, FL 32608, USA; [c] Department of Critical Care, University of Florida, Gainesville, FL, USA; [d] Department of Hospice and Palliative Medicine, University of Florida, Gainesville, FL, USA; [e] Palliative Care Program, North Florida/South Georgia Veterans Health System, Malcom Randall VA Medical Center, University of Florida, 1601 Southwest Archer Road (11F), Gainesville, FL 32608-1197, USA
* Corresponding author.
E-mail address: skitte@ufl.edu

Crit Care Nurs Clin N Am 27 (2015) 315–339
http://dx.doi.org/10.1016/j.cnc.2015.05.010
0899-5885/15/$ – see front matter Published by Elsevier Inc.
ccnursing.theclinics.com

Palliative comes from the Latin root *palliere*, which means to cloak or cover with an outer garment. Keeping this principle in mind when approaching a patient's illness or death, the ultimate goal is to palliate by masking the symptoms of disease to improve the quality of life regardless of how much time remains. Palliative care focuses on a holistic approach to symptom management including physical, psychological, social, and spiritual. For a person to feel well, all aspects of suffering must be addressed to have symptom relief. Treatment should focus on improving quality of life, in line with the patient's goals of care including life prolongation, improved function, or comfort. Informed and shared decision making with respect to each major treatment intervention is critical to the success of management. Transition to comfort care can be considered a viable symptom management strategy if the treatment is overly burdensome.

Health care providers may not be able to cure disease or prevent death, but do have the ability to relieve suffering and improve the quality of life in most patients through aggressive symptom management. Symptom management is a critical component of palliative care consults. In one study involving patients with cancer in an intensive care unit (ICU) setting, 84% of patients receiving palliative consultation had pain.[2] In addition, psychological support is important for patients and their family. Caregivers of patients suffering hospital and ICU deaths are susceptible to heightened and prolonged grief, increased physical and emotional stress, a greater chance of posttraumatic disorder, and a decreased quality of life.[3]

Palliative treatment of patients can occur in conjunction with life-prolonging and curative therapy, or palliative therapy can transition to hospice comfort care if the diagnosis is terminal and prognosis less than 6 months. Hospice care actually results in a mean overall survival benefit of 29 days for many cancers and congestive heart failure (CHF).[4] In brief, palliative care can occur in conjunction with life-prolonging care in critical care settings and results in improved symptom burden, improved patient and caregiver satisfaction, reduced length of stay in the ICU (7.3 days) and hospital, increased hospice referrals, and significant cost savings to the health care system.[5–7]

SYMPTOM ASSESSMENT

Palliative care consultations are often requested to assist with symptom management of a target symptom. When a consultation is requested, providers exchange information about what is most important to accomplish during the visit from the standpoint of the referring clinician. The palliative provider reviews the chart, and often contacts other consultants to gain additional information about treatment options and prognosis when such information requires the expertise of a specialist, such as chemotherapy options from an oncologist. Palliative consults are typically standardized within institutions. Nationally, few validated palliative care quality metrics exist, and overlap with oncology care to include pain assessment, prescription of a bowel regimen with opioids, and advance care planning.[7] Some programs will elect to use symptom score evaluation tools such as the Edmonton Symptom Assessment System and the Palliative Care Symptom Assessment in an attempt to quantify and standardize symptom evaluation.[8,9]

Selection of an evaluation tool can allow for a quantified evaluation and reevaluation of symptoms to enhance treatment, measure impact, improve communication among providers, patients, and families, and identification of comorbid conditions that can affect the outcome of treatments including concomitant depression, anxiety, sleep deprivation, and overall well-being.[8] Symptoms are broken into 2 categories, Pain and Nonpain. A thorough history and physical examination is necessary to determine whether underlying palliative symptoms exist, and the extent to which they affect the patient's overall well-being or activities of daily living.

EVALUATION AND TREATMENT OF PAIN

Pain originates from tissue damage or injury, and in its acute phase leads to protection of the species. Chronic pain results from permanent damage or rewiring of nerves. Pain is subjective, and although diagnostic testing can aid in the determination of its cause, no objective measure or test can quantify pain. Different individuals can experience the same painful stimulus or injury differently because of genetic variance underlying physiologic differences in pain perception and interoperation, or superimposed emotional or spiritual influence. The patient's subjective description can give clues to its origin and aid in selection of a treatment. Pain should be assessed for its onset, location, duration, character, severity, aggravating and relieving factors, timing and treatments tried in the past, functional activities, mood, and sleep impairment. When the patients are not able to relay their pain history, as is often the case in the ICU, symptom assessment comes from nonverbal pain scales, caregiver reports, and subtle physiologic changes including increased heart rate, blood pressure, and respiration.

The Pain Behavior Scale and the Critical-Care Pain Observation Tool have been tested for use in ICU settings.[10] Nonverbal pain scales include the Faces Pain Scale and Wong-Baker FACES Pain Rating Scale. Pain should be treated if anticipated based on the patient's condition or painful interventions, despite the ability of the patient to relay pain subjectively.

- *Somatic pain* is caused by injury to skin, soft tissue, joint, or bone, and is described as aching, stabbing, throbbing, and squeezing.
- *Visceral pain* can be caused by compression, obstruction, infiltration, ischemia, stretching, or inflammation of the viscera, and is described as pressure, cramping, gnawing, and squeezing.
- *Neuropathic pain* results from injury to the peripheral or central nervous system, and is typically burning, shooting, tingling, stabbing, and scalding.[11]

Pharmacologic Treatment of Pain

Pharmacologic options for pain can start with a systematic approach using the modified World Health Organization (WHO) pain ladder, which has proved to be effective in the treatment of pain from all causes, both cancer and noncancer.[12] The WHO first published the pain ladder in 1986 in the handbook titled *Cancer Pain Relief* developed by a group of international experts and translated into 22 languages. Since then, the ladder has guided health care providers worldwide in treating cancer and noncancer pain. In one study of patients with cancer, 87% had complete relief of pain using the WHO guidelines; they have been endorsed as a systematic approach to the treatment of pain by the American Academy of Hospice and Palliative Medicine in their Amplifier Educational Series[11,13] (**Fig. 1**). The most up-to-date pain ladder can be viewed at the WHO Web site (http://www.who.int/cancer/palliative/painladder/en/). After almost 30 years in use, updated treatment ladder guidelines are expected in 2015/2016. The 5 underlying principles of pain management are:

1. For the individual: Dosing of pain medications should be adapted to the individual with a dosage that is adequate to relieve pain and balanced with the side-effect profile.

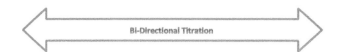

Step 1	Step 2	Step 3	Pain Crisis
(Mild Pain Level 1–3)	(Moderate Pain Level 4–6)	(Severe Pain Level 6–10)	IV/PCa
Non-Opioid analgesics	Weak Opioids	Strong Opioid	Spinal Meds
Acetaminophen	+/- Non-opioid	+/- Non-opioid	Nerve Block
Aspirin	+/- Adjunct	+/- Adjunct	Spinal Stimulator
NSAIDS	Morphine	Long Acting	Surgical Procedures
Ketorolac	Oxycodone	Break Through	+/- Adjunct
	Hydromorphone	Fentanyl Patch	Morphine
	Hydrocodone	Methadone	Hydromorphone
	(+/-) Codeine		Fentanyl

+/- Adjuvant: (Above Non-Opioid Analgesics)

Multipurpose:

Glucocorticoids (Dexamethasone/prednisone)

Antidepressants (TCA, SNRI, SSRI)

Alpha-2-adrenergic agonists (clonidine)

Cannabinoid (THC)

Topical (Lidocaine)

Bowel Obstruction

Anticholinergic (scopolamine)

Somatostatin Analogue (Octreotide)

Neuropathic:

Anticonvulsants (Gabapentin)

Sodium Channel Drugs (lidocaine)

GABA Agonists (clonazepam)

NMDA Inhibitors (ketamine)

Bone Pain:

Bisphosphonates (Pamidronate)

Calcitonin

Holistic Pain Management:

Rehab, Psycho/social/spiritual, Sleep Hygiene, Pharmacologic, Complementary/Alternative/Integrative, Interventional

Fig. 1. Pain management. (*Data from* Vargas-Schaffer G. Is the WHO analgesic ladder still valid. Can Fam Physician 2010;56:514–7; and Takeda F. Relief of cancer pain. Geneva (Switzerland): World Health Organization; 1986.)

2. Attention to detail: Concern for detailed administration of narcotics requires knowledge of the pharmacokinetics, routes, forms, bioavailability, half-life, side effects, and contraindications.
3. By mouth: Oral (or rectal, or nasogastric tube) administration of analgesics is preferred when possible to minimize side effects such as hypotension, often seen in critical care settings, that can result in the undertreatment of pain. Oral medications tend to be well tolerated with fewer side effects, and are safer and less expensive.

4. By the clock: Scheduling medications minimize the chance of breakthrough pain and need for intravenous analgesia, especially in patients who have undergone procedures or surgeries.
5. By the ladder: Prescription should be administered based on pain intensity as rated by a scale of mild, moderate, and severe pain.[13]

Ladder: step 1
Mild pain (score 1–3) should be treated with acetaminophen (Tylenol), Nonsteroidal anti-inflammatory drugs (NSAIDs), and aspirin when possible in a scheduled manner at adequate doses to reduce the level of pain and minimize the need for more aggressive therapy (**Table 1**).

Ladder: step 2
Moderate pain (score 4–6) is treated with a combination of step-1 medications, combined with either weaker/low-dose short-acting opioids or nonopioids as seen in the pain ladder (**Table 2**). Consider if the patient is opioid naïve, and check the weight and renal and liver functions before initiation.

Ladder: step 3
Severe pain: (score 7–10) is treated with escalated doses of stronger and longer-acting opioids with strong consideration of nonopioid adjuncts. Morphine sulfate is the agent of choice in the treatment of severe pain and is a mainstay of palliative

Table 1
Common nonsteroidal anti-inflammatory drugs for mild to moderate pain

| Class | Generic Name | Recommended Initial | | | |
		Onset of Action	Dosing Schedule	Total Daily Dose (mg)	Routes of Administration
Salicylates	Aspirin	2 h	q4–6 h	2400	PO, PR
	Choline magnesium trisalicylate	2 h	q8–12 h	1500	PO
	Salsalate	3–4 d	q8–12 h	3000	PO
P-phenol derivatives	Acetaminophen (paracetamol)	10–60 min	q4–6 h	1300	PO, IV
Propionic acids	Ibuprofen	30–60 min	q4–8 h	1200	PO, IV
	Ketoprofen	<30 min	q6–8 h	200	PO
	Naproxen sodium	1 h	q6–12 h	1250	PO
Acetic acids	Etodolac	2–4 h	q6–8 h	600	PO
	Ketorolac	10 min IM, 2–3 h PO	q4–6 h	120 IV, IM; 40 PO	PO, IV, IM
	Indomethacin	30 min	q8–12 h	100	PO, PR, IV
	Sulindac	3–4 h	q12 h	400	PO
	Diclofenac	30–60 min	q8 h	150	PO
	Nabumetone	4–6 d	Daily	1000	PO
Enolic acids	Piroxicam	1 h	Daily	20	PO
	Meloxicam	4–5 h	Daily	7.5	PO
Selective COX-2 inhibitor	Celecoxib	3 h	Daily to q12 h	200	PO

Abbreviations: COX, cyclooxygenase; IM, intramuscular; IV, intravenous; PO, by mouth; PR, rectally; q, every.
From Goldstein M. Evidence-based practice of palliative care. Philadelphia: Elsevier Saunders; 2013; with permission.

Table 2
Equianalgesic table for adults

Medication	Equianalgesic Dose (for Chronic Dosing)		Usual Starting Doses Adult >50 kg: for Opioid-Naïve Patients (*½ Dose for Elderly, or Severe Renal or Liver Disease)	
	SC/IV	PO	Parenteral	PO
Morphine	10 mg	30 mg	2.5–5 mg SC/IV q3–4 h (*1.25–2.5 mg)	5–15 mg q3–4 h (IR or oral solution) (*2.5–7.5 mg)
Oxycodone	Not available	20 mg	Not available	5–10 mg q3–4 h (*2.5 mg)
Hydromor-phone	1.5 mg	7.5 mg	0.2–0.6 mg SC/IV q2–3 h(*0.2 mg)	1–2 mg q3–4 h (0.5–1 mg)
Codeine	130 mg	200 mg	15–30 mg IM/SC q4 h (*7.5–15 mg) IV contraindicated	30–60 mg q3–4 h (*15–30 mg)
Hydrocodone	Not available	30 mg	Not available	5 mg q3–4 h (*2.5 mg)
Methadone (see text for dosing conversions)	½ oral dose 2 mg PO methadone +1 mg parenteral methadone	24-h oral morphine — <30 mg / 31–99 mg / 100–299 mg / 300–499 mg / 500–999 mg / 1000–1200 mg / >1200 mg — Oral morphine: methadone ratio — 2:1 / 4:1 / 8:1 / 12:1 / 15:1 / 20:1 / Consider consult	1.25–2.5 mg q8 h (*1.25 mg)	2.5–5 mg q8 h (*1.25–2.5 mg)

		24-h oral MS dose	Initial patch dose	25–50 µg IM/IV q1–3 h (*12.5–25 µg)	Transdermal patch 12.5 µg/h q72 h (use with caution in opioid-naïve and unstable patients because of 12-h delay in onset and offset)
Fentanyl (see text for dosing Conversions)	100 µg single dose (T$_{1/2}$ and duration of parenteral doses variable)	30–59 mg 60–134 mg 135–224 mg 225–314 mg 315–404 mg	12.5 µg/h 25 µg/h 50 µg/h 75 µg/h 100 µg/h	—	
Not recommended	—	—			—
Meperidine	75–100 mg	300 mg		75 mg SC/IM q2–3 h (*25–50 mg) Generally not recommended	Not recommended

Developed by palliative care programs at the University of Rochester Medical Center, ViaHealth, Unity Health, and Excellus BlueCross/BlueShield.
Abbreviations: IR, immediate release; SC, subcutaneous.
Adapted from Quill TE. Guide to alleviating physical and psychological pain in patients with serious of life-threatening conditions. 2012; with permission.

care. Other practical factors guide prescribing, including cost, availability, and the patient's health literacy with complex medical regimens. Side effects should be anticipated and a bowel regimen for constipation prescribed. Side effects such as nausea, pruritus, and sedation typically diminish over a week.

Ladder: step 4

Severe uncontrolled pain or pain crisis is not uncommon in hospital settings in caring for patients with life-limiting illness and at the end of life. A modified version of the WHO pain ladder accounts for this, with options for intravenous administration of pain medication, use of a patient-controlled analgesia (PCA) pump, nerve blocks, epidurals, and spinal stimulators.[12]

Intravenous pain control is rapid, predictable, and useful in patients when oral administration is not an option. Intravenous use should be limited because of its disadvantages, including the cost and complexity of continuous administration; even in palliative care or hospice settings, alternative routes of administration are preferred.

Intravenous PCA provides superior postoperative analgesia and improves patient satisfaction.[2] In nonsurgical patients, this can be considered to achieve patient-titrated pain control to obtain a 24-hour total of narcotic necessary to achieve pain relief and conversion into a longer-acting option for deescalation of care when clinically appropriate in alert patients. In one study involving patients with cancer in ICU settings, 84% receiving palliative consultation had pain; the most common treatment recommendations included change of opioid (99%), starting opioids (44%), drug rotation (34%), change of dose (20%), adding steroids (70%), and treatment of side effects including addition of antiemetics (79%) and starting a bowel regimen (72%).[3]

Palliative sedation is considered in rare circumstances of uncontrolled severe pain and refractory terminal symptoms, when death is imminent. In one study, palliative sedation was used more for patients who suffered from terminal delirium (62%) and dyspnea (47%), compared with uncontrolled pain (28%). It was not associated with hastening of death.[14] Palliative sedation should only be considered following shared medical decision making with the patient or their health care surrogate, and after multidisciplinary review. Some institutions may require informed consent based on local policy.

Key Points in Pain Management

- Titration. The WHO pain ladder can move up or down as symptoms worsen or improve based on disease progression, treatment, or other physiologic factors. Pain control is a balance between symptom relief and side-effect profile.
- Rotation or conversion. At least 10% of patients will experience persistent pain and/or intolerable side effects to a particular opioid, and providers should consider rotation to a different opioid. In addition, conversion is common in hospital and critical care settings when route of administration and formulary can change from outpatient settings.
  - Calculate the equianalgesic dose from a table or on-line calculator tool. Automatically reduce the dose 25% to 50% less than calculated dose. Assess response frequently and titrate accordingly. See the on-line calculator for conversion and additional information: www.globalrph.com/
  - Exception: Fentanyl (Duragesic transdermal) does not require dose reduction. Continuation of the original medication for 24 hours while fentanyl reaches its therapeutic level is necessary.

- ○ *Exception:* Methadone hydrochloride (Diskets Dispersible; Dolophine; Methadone HCl Intensol) requires 75% to 90% dose reduction given its long and unpredictable patient-dependent half-life. It is an excellent and inexpensive pain reliever, but caution must be used given the multiple drug interactions and potential to prolong the QT interval.[15]
- Breakthrough. Most patients started on long-acting opioids for severe pain will require breakthrough pain medications. Principals of breakthrough pain management are as follows:
  - ○ In the ICU or hospital setting, intravenous breakthrough pain medication is typically 50% of a 1-hour dose given intravenously every 15 minutes. Oral pain breakthrough administration is typically 10% of the 24-hour dose given orally every 2 hours.[10]
- Side effects. Analgesics, specifically opiates, should be prescribed with careful attention to balancing desirable treatment effects against those side effects that may be perceived as adverse to the patient and caregiver. Typical side effects of opioid medications include constipation, nausea, somnolence, myoclonus, seizures, respiratory depression, hypogonadism, and sleep-related breathing disorder. Proper selection of opiate type, dose, and schedule should be based on underlying comorbidities and may improve tolerance of side effects. Specifically, patients with renal impairment, hepatic insufficiency, or on concomitant sedating medications may be at higher risk for oversedation or respiratory depression.

Anticipatory treatment of predictable side effects includes concomitant administration of stool softeners at the time of treatment initiation. Intravenous administration is often accompanied by nausea in opioid-naïve individuals and pruritis. Coadministration of an antiemetic agent and antihistamine respectively reduces this response. Hyperalgesia is a rare physiologic phenomenon whereby opioid exposure lowers the threshold for pain and leads to hyperalgesia in response to stimuli without clear progression of pathologic condition. Symptoms can be accompanied by confusion, tremor, and skin sensitivity. Opioid rotation or nonopioid intervention should also be considered.[10]

Nonopioid Analgesics and Adjuvant Analgesia

The WHO pain ladder appropriately uses nonopioid analgesics first for mild pain. For more intense levels of pain, clinicians can use nonnarcotics as an adjunct to decrease the need for high doses of opioids, given the risk/benefit profile of opioid analgesics. Obtaining a thorough history to determine the type of pain can assist with nonopioid selection. Typical options (**Table 3**) include.

- Acetaminophen (Tylenol, Panadol) can relieve mild pain similarly to aspirin but has no anti-inflammatory effects. It is available in rectal and intravenous form, but dosing by any route is limited by liver toxicity.
- NSAIDs have excellent analgesic and anti-inflammatory properties, and intravenous forms are available in the inpatient setting. Use may be limited by renal dysfunction and gastrointestinal side effects.
- Of the steroids, glucocorticoids are the strongest anti-inflammatory medications, with multiple palliative beneficial side effects including appetite stimulation, relief of nausea, pain relief, and euphoria or sense of well-being. This combination is especially beneficial to patients with late-stage illness associated with lung disease, cancer, or pain.[10] Consider empiric treatment with an H2 blocker or proton-pump inhibitor in the event of increased stomach acid

Table 3
Adjuvant analgesics

Drug Class	Subclass	Examples	Comments
Multipurpose Analgesics			
Glucocorticoids	NA	Dexamethasone Prednisone	Used for bone pain, neuropathic pain, lymphedema pain, headache, bowel obstruction
Antidepressants	Tricyclics	Desipramine, amitriptyline	Used for opioid-refractory neuropathic pain First if comorbid depression; secondary amine compounds (eg, desipramine) have fewer side effects and may be preferred
	SNRIs	Duloxetine, milnacipran	Good evidence in some conditions but overall less than tricyclics; however, better side-effect profile; often tried first
	Other	Bupropion	Limited evidence but less sedating, and often tried early when fatigue or somnolence is a problem
α2-Adrenergic	NA	Tizanidine, clonidine	Seldom used systemically because of side effects, But tizanidine is preferred for a trial; clonidine is used in neuraxial analgesia
Cannabinoid	NA	THC/cannabidiol, nabilone, THC	Good evidence in cancer pain for THC/cannabidiol; limited evidence for other commercially available compounds
Topical agents	Anesthetic	Lidocaine patch Local anesthetic creams	NA —
	Capsaicin	8% patch; 0.25%, 0.75% creams	High-concentration patch indicated for postherpetic neuralgia

Used for Neuropathic Pain

Multipurpose drugs	As above	As above	As above
Anticonvulsants	Gabapentinoids	Gabapentin, pregabalin	Used first for opioid-refractory neuropathic pain unless comorbid depression; may be multipurpose considering evidence in postsurgical pain; both drugs act at the N-type calcium channel in the CNS, but responsive to one or the other varies
	Other	Oxcarbazepine, lamotrigine, topiramate, lacosamide, divalproex, carbamazepine, phenytoin	Limited evidence for all examples listed; newer drugs preferred because of less side-effect liability, but individual variation is wide; all are considered for opioid-refractory neuropathic pain if antidepressants and gabapentinoids are ineffective
Sodium channel drugs	Sodium channel Blockers	Mexiletine	Good evidence for IV lidocaine
		IV lidocaine	—

Multipurpose Analgesics

Sodium channel drugs (cont.)	Sodium channel modulator	Lacosamide	New anticonvulsant with limited evidence of analgesic effects
GABA agonists	$GABA_A$ agonist	Clonazepam	Limited evidence, but used for neuropathic pain with anxiety
	$GABA_B$ agonist	Baclofen	Evidence in trigeminal neuralgia is the basis for trials in other types of neuropathic pain
N-Methyl-D-aspartate inhibitors	NA	Ketamine, memantine, others	Limited evidence for ketamine, but positive experience for IV use in advanced illness or a pain crisis; little evidence for oral drugs

(continued on next page)

Table 3
(continued)

Drug Class	Subclass	Examples	Comments
Used for Bone Pain			
Bisphosphonates	NA	Pamidronate, ibandronate, clodronate	Good evidence; like the NSAIDs or glucocorticoids, usually considered first-line therapy; also reduces other adverse skeletal-related events; concern about osteonecrosis of the jaw and renal insufficiency; may limit use
Calcitonin	NA	NA	Limited evidence but usually well tolerated
Radiopharmaceuticals	NA	Strontium-89, samarium-153	Good evidence, but limited use because of bone marrow effects and need for expertise
Used for Bowel Obstruction			
Anticholinergic drugs	NA	Scopolamine (hyoscine) compounds, glycopyrrolate	Along with a glucocorticoid, considered first-line adjuvant for nonsurgical bowel obstruction
Somatostatin analogue	NA	Octreotide	Along with a glucocorticoid, considered first-line adjuvant for nonsurgical bowel obstruction

Abbreviations: CNS, central nervous system; GABA, γ-aminobutyric acid; IV, intravenous; NA, not applicable; NSAID, nonsteroidal anti-inflammatory drug; SNRI, serotonin norepinephrine reuptake inhibitor; THC, tetrahydrocannabinol.

From Portenoy RK. Treatment of cancer pain. Lancet 2011;377(9784):49; with permission.

secretion. Caution must be used in long-term use given the side effects of immunosuppression and hypoadrenalism.

- Analgesic antidepressants can have a benefit in chronic pain, and can improve pain independent of depression or effect on mood by modulating monoamines including norepinephrine, serotonin, and dopamine, to play a role in analgesia. Tricyclic antidepressants (TCAs) are inexpensive and are used for neuropathic pain, headache suppression, and insomnia. Serotonin norepinephrine reuptake inhibitors (SNRIs) tend to be less effective than the older TCAs but with a better side-effect profile, often leading to their use first. Limited evidence of pain treatment exists with selective serotonin reuptake inhibitors (SSRIs), but treatment of depression and anxiety may improve the psychological component of pain and can be considered.[11]

- For neuropathic pain, anticonvulsants such as gabapentin (Neurontin) and pregabalin (Lyrica) are first-line medications, and may be beneficial in combination with opioid-refractory pain conditions. γ-Aminobutyric acid agonists, such as clonazepam, may have a role in decreasing neuropathic pain and pain with underlying anxiety. These agents, however, may be associated with increased somnolence and sedation.

- Benzodiazepines have multiple beneficial treatment effects in the palliative care setting including sedation, relief of anxiety, pain adjunct for muscle relaxation, and nausea, and in the treatment of delirium, alcohol withdrawal, and insomnia.

- Muscle relaxants can help alleviate musculoskeletal pain and spasms and reduce spasticity in a variety of neurologic conditions. These agents may increase somnolence and sedation.

- For bone pain, bisphosphonates should be considered as a pain adjunct to reduce pain, and as an analgesic to manage metastatic bone pain. Bisphosphonates can be used for 12 weeks during a trial for pain control with close evaluation of dental health before implementation.[16]

- Cannabinoids have shown benefit in the treatment of cancer-related pain, but evidence is limited for the commercially available compounds. Several states have approved the use of medical marijuana available from natural sources rather than commercial products. Side effects may include increased somnolence.

- For topical analgesia, lidocaine patch (Lidoderm) for topical pain, gel for preprocedural analgesia, or liquid for pain associated with mucositis or chronic radiation esophagitis can be considered. High-concentration capsaicin, available topically, can improve neuropathic pain conditions but requires frequent dosing. The topical NSAID diclofenac (Voltaren, Cataflam, Zorvolex, Zipsor) is useful for musculoskeletal pain when patients cannot tolerate systemic NSAIDs because of gastrointestinal side effects or renal impairment.

- Ketamine (Ketalar) has a limited role in acute sickle cell pain crisis or advanced illness. Side effects include emergence reactions and hallucinations.

Nonpharmacologic Pain Management

Advanced therapies, including surgical debulking, catheters to relieve pleural or abdominal malignant fluid accumulation, esophageal and pulmonary stents, anesthesia pain block, vertebroplasty, chemotherapy, and radiation, can be palliative if the intent is to relieve symptom burden, even in patients who have forgone curative therapy. Advanced therapies carry additional cost and potential treatment burden, and should be carefully considered after more traditional therapies have been implemented. Advanced procedures can often be symptom relieving, even in terminal patients whose goal of care is comfort. Interdisciplinary treatment plans are useful in complex critical care patients with advanced disease and unrelieved pain. Lastly, sleep hygiene has recently been discussed as playing a significant role in the modulation and perception of pain.

NONPAIN SYMPTOM MANAGEMENT
Pulmonary

Dyspnea is a sensation of air hunger or shortness of breath that may be accompanied by increased work of breathing and chest tightness, causing anxiety and discomfort. Although it is related to respiratory rate, oxygen saturation, and hypercapnia, its measurement is subjective. As with pain, subjective measure of shortness of breath can be assessed in a quantitative evaluation using the same Edmonton Symptom Assessment System used to measure pain, Dyspnea severity measurement can help monitor the impact of therapeutic success. Shortness of breath can be caused by multiple disease entities and physiologic conditions. Determining the underlying cause by thorough history, physical, laboratory, and radiographic testing can aid the success of treatment of the symptoms if correcting the underlying condition is possible. Noninvasive, nonpharmacologic treatment includes blowing fan air in the face, caregiver support, repositioning, pulmonary and cardiac rehabilitation, cool temperature, and careful planning of activities to include assistance and pacing. Causes of dyspnea and treatments are outlined in **Table 4**.[16] As with any palliative symptom, goals of care determine the extent of workup, invasiveness of treatment, and risk versus benefit of treatment.

Oxygen

In many patients, the use of supplemental oxygen may serve to enhance the quality of life by decreasing air hunger or work of breathing. Oxygen can be delivered by nasal

Table 4 Causes and treatments of dyspnea	
All-cause	Opioids: hydrocodone 2.5–5 mg PO q4 h, morphine sulfate 2.5–5 mg PO q4 h, oxycodone 5 mg PO q4, hydromorphone 1–2 mg PO q4 h
Anemia	Blood transfusion, iron/vitamin supplementation, erythropoietin
Anxiety	Adjunct anxiolytic (benzodiazepine, SSRI)
Bronchospasm	Albuterol, ipratropium, steroids
Cancer	Chemoradiation, pulmonary stenting, tumor debulking
Congestive heart failure	Diuretic, vasodilators, inotrope, dialysis, fluid/salt restriction
Chronic Illness (HIV, ALS, CVA)	Similar treatment as above; see Palliative Care Fast Facts: http://www.eperc.mcw.edu/EPERC/FastFactsandConcepts
COPD	Nebulized saline, guaifenesin
Effusions:	Thoracentesis, chemical or mechanical pleurodesis, tunneled palliative pleural catheter
Infection	Antibiotics
Terminal secretions	Scopolamine, atropine drops, glycopyrrolate

Abbreviations: ALS, amyotrophic lateral sclerosis; COPD, chronic obstructive pulmonary disease; CVA, cerebrovascular accident; HIV, human immunodeficiency virus; SSRI, selective serotonin reuptake inhibitor.

cannula, face mask, High-Flow Nasal Cannula, or noninvasive ventilation (NIV) support, commonly referred to as continuous positive airway pressure or bilevel positive airway pressure. Supplemental oxygen is administered if it provides subjective improvement and is tolerated. Noninvasive ventilatory support that provides supplemental oxygen has the additional benefit of reducing the work of breathing in CHF, or in patients with fluid retention. It is also used to improve the quality of sleep in obesity hypoventilation or obstructive sleep apnea. In select cases, NIV may be considered a palliative treatment, particularly when the underlying issue is short-lived; that is, the need for diuresis. However, because of mask discomfort, risk of pressure ulceration, gastric distension, aspiration, claustrophobia, and anxiety, application should be reserved for alert patients who are capable of tolerating brief intervals of 2 to 6 hours of therapy. Additional consideration should be made regarding advanced directives and the use of a mechanical device to prolong life before initiation. Generally speaking, NIV should not be initiated as palliative therapy for the actively dying patient (ie, hours to days).

Dialysis

The initiation of palliative hemodialysis in end-of-life patients with renal failure to manage respiratory symptoms remains an acceptable practice following shared medical decision making and a discussion regarding the goals of care. In select patients, hemodialysis can improve work of breathing and mentation, allowing patients to participate in activities of daily living in the short term. Risks of hemodialysis include complications related to the placement of a venous catheter, infection, fatigue, bleeding, hypotension, and cardiac arrest. Alternatives should be carefully explored and weighed against the goals of initiating dialysis therapy. Once discontinued, mean survival is typically 1 to 2 weeks.[17] At the end of life, opiates such as fentanyl and methadone may be better tolerated in patients with renal failure, reducing the incidence of seizures and myoclonic jerking.[18]

Opioids

Opioids are the first-line pharmacologic treatment in patients with dyspnea associated with advanced disease. Opioids are used successfully in patients with chronic obstructive pulmonary disease, CHF, and in patients with cancer.[19] No specific opioid has been shown to be superior in the treatment of dyspnea, as each has a similar mechanism of action. Scheduled medications may be necessary in the setting of chronic dyspnea. Caution should be used to observe for sedation and efficacy. If treatment is not successful, it should be weaned and discontinued. Refractory dyspnea can often be successfully treated with adjunct benzodiazepines in palliative patients.[20] Typical opioid medications and starting doses are listed in **Table 2**.[19] Consideration of long-acting sustained relief preparations in refractory dyspnea, chronic dyspnea, or opioid-tolerant individuals. Terminal secretions result from secretions pooling in the back of the throat and has been referred to as the "death rattle." Patients are usually unconscious and unaware of the noise and secretions. Family education, soft background music, and reassurance of the normal dying process is necessary, in addition to pharmacologic treatments including opioids and medications to dry secretions.

Compassionate Withdrawal of Artificial Life Support

Compassionate withdrawal of artificial life support (formerly called withdrawal of care) involves careful discussion and decision making between interdisciplinary teams, patients, and families while adhering to institutional policies and procedures. No one protocol is superior, but any approach should be standardized to allow for patient comfort, anticipation and relief of pain, agitation, dyspnea, and terminal secretions while providing emotional and spiritual support to the family. Leaving the endotracheal tube in place and ventilator weaning are both reasonable approaches.

Gastrointestinal Symptoms

Nausea, vomiting, anorexia, dysphagia, bowel obstruction, and constipation are common symptoms in palliative patients. Given the diversity of symptoms, etiology, and treatment, a through history and physical examination is imperative in determining the cause and best treatment plan.

Dysphagia can result from myopathies, neuromuscular disorders, anatomic disease of the nasopharynx, and systemic disease (**Table 5**).[19]

Nausea and Vomiting

Nausea and vomiting are common and debilitating symptoms that can result in decreased quality of life, dehydration, and weight loss. As with pain, careful history and physical examination to determine the underlying cause of symptoms aid in prevention and treatment of distressing symptoms. Examples of treatment for prevention of overreaction include scheduling a stool-softener bowel regimen at the time of starting opioids, and coadministration of an antiemetic with intravenous narcotic in opioid-naïve individuals and chemotherapy patients to prevent nausea and vomiting, dehydration, and electrolyte disturbances. Potential causes of nausea include intracerebral causes (tumor, increased intracerebral pressure, anxiety, pain), vestibular system, chemoreceptor trigger zone (medications such as opioids, chemotherapy, and antibiotics, metabolic organ failure, and electrolyte disturbance), and gastrointestinal/peripheral track causes (medications, tumor, radiation, constipation, obstruction, gag reflex, cough).[21] A summary of the treatment approach is outlined in **Tables 6** and **7**.

Constipation

Constipation can result from medications, poor diet, and dehydration leading to pain, nausea, obstruction, and hospitalization. Common medications that cause constipation include opioids, anticholinergics, iron/calcium supplementation, and calcium-channel blockers. Educating patients and families that most constipation medications are safe, inexpensive, can be taken daily, and are available without prescription allows them to self-manage their bowel regimens. Consider increasing doses when ineffective before adding additional agents. The aggressiveness of the regimen often depends on the patient's regular bowel habits, duration since bowel movement, ability to take oral medications, and associated severity of symptom such as pain or vomiting. Suppositories, enemas, and manual disimpaction can be used as second-line treatments given their invasiveness if oral treatment fails.[19] In patients suffering from opiate-induced constipation refractory to other methods, an option is oral naloxone (intravenous preparation administered orally), although this is not approved by the Food and Drug Administration. Oral naloxone reverses the bowel dysmotility and constipation induced by opiate use but binds less than 5% of systemic opiate, so that patients do not have to discontinue administration of oral medication for pain (**Table 8**).[22]

Anorexia and Cachexia

Anorexia is a common problem associated with terminal and chronic illnesses. Its cause is multifactorial, including loss of appetite, decreased intake, and abnormal metabolism, which result in loss of muscle mass, hypoalbuminemia, and functional impairment. Treatment should involve a through history and physical examination to identify reversible causes termed secondary nutrition impact syndrome (SNIS). SNIS

Table 5 Causes of dysphagia	
	Treatment
Myopathies	
GERD	PPI, GERD diet, elevation head of bed
Radiation damage	Magic Mouth Wash
Neoplasm	Stent, DHT/NG, debulking, chemoradiation
Achalasia	Dilatation
Scleroderma	Dilatation
Esophagitis	PPI, treatment of infection
Infectious Etiology/Injury	
Sinusitis	Allergy medication, antibiotics
Thrush	Nystatin, clotrimazole, fluconazole
Viral infection	Acyclovir
Injury	DHT, NG, PEG, TPN
Neuromuscular Disorders	
CVA, nerve damage, Parkinson, MS, myasthenia gravis, dementias	Speech therapy for the disorder, specific diet, aspiration precautions, safe diet (puree, thickened liquids), comfort care feedings to taste/moisten mouth, advanced artificial hydration and nutrition via DHT, NG, PEG, TPN
ENT	
Dental caries, poorly fitting or lack of dentures, allergies, nasal drying from oxygen, mucositis from damage or dryness	Dental hygiene, replace dentures, humidified oxygen, salivary substitute, sugar-free gum, oral gel, pilocarpine, combination mouthwash (topical lidocaine, nystatin, hydrocortisone, loperamide, opioids, doxepin)
Systemic	
Nutritional deficiencies, dehydration, thyroid disorders	Rehydration, popsicles, sips, sponge sticks, artificial hydration, nutrition. Scant evidence supports the use of artificial hydration and nutrition in patients with advance disease

Abbreviations: ENT, ear/nose/throat; DHT, dobhoff tube; GERD, gastroesophageal reflux disease; MS, multiple sclerosis; NG, nasogastric tube; PEG, polyethylene glycol; PPI, proton-pump inhibitor; TPN, total parenteral nutrition.

includes physiologic problems associated with taste, eating, constipation, nausea, vomiting, pain, delirium, or dyspnea.[23] Artificial nutrition and hydration can be considered depending on goals of care. Anorexia and cachexia are physiologic manifestations that accompany the dying process. Offering a taste of food or mouth moistening is often sufficient, and can be satisfying to anorexic patients. Forcing more food and liquid may prove more harmful than beneficial. Cachexia is the irreversible loss of muscle mass that cannot be reversed nutritionally despite adequate caloric intake, and is a poor prognostic indicator. Pharmacologic treatment can include[19]:

- Megestrol acetate (Megace; Megace ES): start 400 mg by mouth daily, increase to 600 to 800 mg/d at 2 weeks
- Olanzapine (Zyprexa): 5 mg by mouth daily
- Corticosteroids: prednisone, 20 to 40 mg by mouth daily or dexamethasone, 2 to 8 mg by mouth daily

Table 6
Cause-based classification of nausea and vomiting

Clinical Syndrome	General Cause	Features	Receptor Pathways	Treatment
Chemical	*Medications*: Opioids, digoxin, anticonvulsants, antibiotics, antifungals, cytotoxics, SSRIs, iron *Toxins*: Ischemic bowel, infection, tumor products *Metabolic*: Renal failure, liver failure, hypercalcemia, hyponatremia, ketoacidosis	Drug toxicity, associated underlying disease, constant nausea, variable vomiting	Stimulation of $D_2 \pm$ 5-HT3 in CTZ Chemotherapy stimulates serotonin release in GI tract, 5-HT3 on vagus Chemotherapy stimulates NK_1 receptors in brain	Check drug levels, stop offending drug Treat underlying cause Haloperidol or phenothiazine 5-HT3 antagonists for CINV and radiation-related NK for CINV
Impaired gastric emptying	*Medications*: Opioids, tricyclic antidepressants, phenothiazines, anticholinergics Ascites Hepatosplenomegaly Autonomic dysfunction Tumor infiltration	Epigastric fullness or pain, early satiety, flatulence, reflux, hiccups, large-volume emesis	Gastric mechanoreceptors stimulate vagal afferents to the VC Additional receptors: H1, Achm	Treat underlying cause(s) Prokinetics (metoclopramide) Large-volume paracentesis
Visceral causes	Peritoneal carcinomatosis Bowel obstruction Gastroenteritis, gastritis Constipation, fecal impaction Stretched liver capsule Ureteral distension	Diffuse, dull aching or crampy abdominal pain that may radiate to shoulder, abdomen	Gut/serosal mechanoreceptors stimulate vagus	Aggressive bowel regimen Reduce acid secretions with H_2-blocker or PPI Medical or surgical management of obstruction Corticosteroids may reduce tumor mass
Cortical	Increased intracranial pressure: intracranial tumor, cerebral infarct, infection, bleed Meningeal irritation Leptomeningeal carcinomatosis Anxiety, pain	Headache, visual changes, focal neurologic deficits	Direct stimulation of receptors in vomiting center (HT2, Achm, H1) via intracerebral projections	Treat reversible cause Benzodiazepines Corticosteroids may reduce tumor mass
Vestibular	Medications Motion sickness Labyrinthine disorders	Symptoms correspond to position change, vertigo	Stimulation of Achm and histamine in the vestibular apparatus	Stop offending drug Meclizine Antihistamines

Abbreviations: 5-HT, serotonin; Achm, anticholinergic muscarinic; CINV, chemotherapy-induced nausea and vomiting; CTZ, chemoreceptor trigger zone; GI, gastrointestinal; NK, neurokinin; SSRI, selective serotonin reuptake inhibitor; VC, vomiting center.

Adapted from Glare P, Pereira G, Kristjanson LJ, et al. Systematic review of the efficacy of antiemetics in the treatment of nausea in patients with far-advanced cancer. Support Care Cancer 2004;12(6):432–40; and Goldstein M. Evidence-based practice of palliative care. Philadelphia: Elsevier Saunders; 2013.

Table 7
Common receptor-specific therapies for nausea and emesis not related to chemotherapy

Class	Drug	Receptor	Site	Dosing	Side Effects
Dopamine antagonists	Promethazine	D2, Achm, H1	CTZ	PO/IV: 12.5–25 mg q6 h PR: 25 mg q6 h	Sedation, orthostatic hypotension, extrapyramidal side effects
	Prochlorperazine	D2	CTZ	PO/IV: 5–10 g q6 h PR: 25 mg q6 h	
	Chlorpromazine	D2	CTZ	PO: 10–25 mg q4 h IV: 25–50 mg q4 h PR: 50–100 mg q4 h	
	Haloperidol	D2	CTZ	PO/subcutaneously: 0.5–5 mg Q8–12 h	
Prokinetic	Metoclopramide	D2, 5-HT3, Achm	CTZ, GI tract	PO/IV/SC: 10–20 mg q6 h	Avoid in complete GI obstruction
Serotonin antagonist	Ondansetron	5-HT3	GI tract, CTZ, VC	PO/ODT/IV: 4–8 mg q4–8 h	Constipation, diarrhea, fatigue, headache, possible QTc prolongation
Antihistamines	Diphenhydramine	H1	Vestibular	PO/IV/SC: 25–50 mg q6 h	Dry mouth, drowsiness, confusion, urinary retention
	Meclizine	H1	Vestibular	PO: 12.5–50 mg q6 h	Dry mouth, drowsiness, blurred vision
Anticholinergics	Hyoscyamine	Achm	Vestibular	PO/SL: 0.125–0.25 mg q4 h IV/SC: 0.25–0.5 mg q4 h	Dry mouth, blurred vision, urinary retention constipation, confusion
	Scopolamine	Achm	Vestibular	Transdermal patch: 1–3 applied q72 h Gel: 0.25% applied topically q4–6 h	
Antidepressant	Mirtazapine	5-HT3	GI tract, CTZ, VC	PO: 15–45 mg at night	Dizziness, blurred vision, sedation, somnolence, malaise increased appetite, weight gain, dry mouth, constipation, vivid dreams
Atypical antipsychotic	Olanzapine	D2, Achm 5-HT3, H1	GI tract, CTZ, VC	PO: 2.5–10 mg q24 h	Increased appetite, weight gain, hyperglycemia, sedation, reduced seizure threshold, increased serum lipids

Abbreviations: Achm, anticholinergic muscarinic; CTZ, chemoreceptor trigger zone; D1, D2, dopamine receptors; GI, gastrointestinal; ODT, oral dissolving tablet; SL, sublingual; VC, vomiting center.
Reprinted from Goldstein M. Evidence-based practice of palliative medicine. Elsevier; 2013. p. 143; with permission.

Table 8
Commonly used laxatives for opioid-induced constipation

Group	Action	Agents	Latency	Side Effects/Cautions
Bulking agents	Increase fecal bulk, retain fluid in gut lumen	Psyllium seed, bran, methylcellulose	Days	Bloating, flatulence, abdominal pain Risk of exacerbating constipation if inadequate fluid intake Generally not recommended in patients with advanced illness
Osmotics	Draw and maintain water within gut lumen, increase fluid secretion in small bowel	Magnesium sulfate (eg, Milk of Magnesia, magnesium citrate, Epsom salts)	1–3 h	Abdominal cramping, watery stools, dehydration, hypermagnesemia, hypocalcemia, hyperphosphatemia Not recommended in patients with cardiac and renal disease
		Lactulose	24–48 h	Bloating, flatulence, colic, sweet taste, hypokalemia, hypernatremia, lactic acidosis, acid-base disturbance
		Polyethylene glycol (eg, MiraLax)	0.5–1 h	Nausea, abdominal cramping, bloating, diarrhea, flatulence, fecal incontinence Aspiration into lungs can result in pulmonary edema
Stimulants	Alter intestinal permeability, stimulates myenteric plexus to induce peristalsis	Anthroquinones; senna, cacara	6–12 h	Abdominal cramping, colic melanosis coli with chronic use
		Biscodyl	6–12	Abdominal cramping, electrolyte imbalance

Surfactants	Docusate sodium	Detergents, lubricate and soften stools	12–72 h	Limited efficacy, not recommended as solo agent
Suppositories	Glycerin	Reflex evacuation through direct stimulation	0.25–1 h	Rectal irritation, ineffective if feces located higher in colon
	Biscodyl		0.25–1 h	Rectal irritation, ineffective if feces located higher in colon
Enemas	Saline, sodium phosphate	Draw water into lumen	0.5–1 h	Dehydration, hypocalcemia, hyperphosphatemia; Not recommended in patients with renal disease
	Tap water, soapsuds, Mineral oil	Distention, facilitation peristalsis	0.5–1 h	Repeated tap water enemas may lead to fluid and electrolyte abnormalities; Soapsuds have been associated with chemical colitis
Opioid receptor	Naloxone	Competitive opioid antagonist	0.5–4 h	Opioid withdrawal; not indicated in most patients
	Methylnaltrexone	Selective peripheral opioid antagonist	0.5–4 h	Abdominal cramps, nausea, soft stools, diarrhea, flatulence, nausea; Contraindicated in setting of bowel obstruction

From Goldstein. Evidence-based practice of palliative medicine. Elsevier; 2013. p. 132; with permission.

- Eicosapentaenoic acid, 3 g by mouth daily
- Medroxyprogesterone (Depo-Provera, Provera, Depo-Provera contraceptive), 200 to 400 mg per day
- L-Carnitine (Carnitor), 4 g daily
- Cannabinoids (Dronabinol, Marinol), 2.5 mg by mouth twice a day (20 mg/d maximum)
- Thalidomide (Thalomid), 200 mg by mouth daily

Fatigue

Fatigue is a persistent sense of tiredness that interferes with function and quality of life caused by multiple factors, including:

- Illness
- Anorexia/cachexia
- Treatment
- Terminal conditions
- Psychosocial causes
- Chronic inflammation
- Depression
- Sleep disturbance
- Pain

Treatment includes addressing underlying causes such as anemia, malnutrition, depression, and pain. A review of the literature, including a 2010 Cochrane review, found scant evidence of pharmacologic effectiveness in the treatment of fatigue in palliative patients.[24] Some possible treatment options include methylphenidate (Concerta, Metadate CD, Metadate ER, Methylin, Methylin ER, Quillivant XR, Ritalin, Ritalin LA, Ritalin SR), amantadine (Symmetrel), modafinil (Provigil), and corticosteroids.[19] Nonpharmacologic treatment such as physical therapy to conserve energy may be beneficial.

Bowel Obstruction

Bowel obstruction results from multiple causes and can at times be conservatively managed with nasogastric tube placement and bowel rest. In terminal illness, obstruction can be fatal, and decompressive ostomy surgery can be considered depending on the condition and goals of care. Noninvasive management of malignant bowel obstruction includes adding anticholinergic agents such as scopolamine to decrease secretions and colicky pain, antidopaminergic agents such as Haldol to help with nausea, and steroids to decrease bowel edema and inflammation. Advanced treatment can include a trial of octreotide (Sandostatin, Sandostatin LAR Depot) that decreases gastric secretions, intestinal motility, and blood flow, and increased the quality of life in 56% of patients, with no adverse side effects.[25,26] In patients who suffer from recurrent adhesive-related small bowel obstruction, who are not surgical candidates, preventive and therapeutic measures may include abdominal or visceral massage therapy.[27]

Mood Disorders

Mood disorders such as anxiety and depression are common in the general population (8.9%) and in patients with advanced illness (12.9%).[2] Given its prevalence, it is important to screen patients with advanced illness for mood disorders, as physical symptoms from the underlying illness may confound the presentation. Screening for mood disorders is included in the previously mentioned palliative care symptom assessment tools. Because depression and anxiety can result from organic illness, a diagnosis of mood disorder is based on exclusion. A personal and family history of psychiatric illness can aid in diagnosis. Treatment options for depression and anxiety include psychotherapy, cognitive-behavioral therapy, music, relaxation, mindfulness/meditation, art, exercise, sleep hygiene, and pharmacologic therapy. Pharmacologic therapy options for depression include the psychostimulants methylphenidate and dextroamphetamine (Adderall, Adderall XR) in patients with a prognosis of less than 6 months, and for a prognosis longer than 6 months typical treatment options include SSRIs, SNRIs, bupropion (Wellbutrin; Wellbutrin XL; Wellbutrin SR; Zyban), mirtazapine (Remeron; Remeron Soltab), and TCAs. For anxiety, pharmacologic treatment options for patients with serious illness include anxiolytics, SSRIs, benzodiazepines, trazodone (Desyrel), and gabapentin.[2]

Delirium

Delirium is a common presentation to the emergency room (ER) otherwise known as altered mental status, and is discussed in the article elsewhere in this issue by Solberg on Palliative Care in the ER.

Psychosocial and Spiritual Pain

The grief experienced with disease, illness, or the prospect of death may manifest as a struggle with one's self-image, spirituality, or religious beliefs. Patients may experience guilt, feelings of abandonment, fear, anxiety, or ambivalence, all of which may manifest as pain or other physical symptoms qualified as suffering. Careful history and review that includes the assessment of pain and the value of spirituality in addition to feelings of hope, meaning, and spiritual well-being may provide important avenues for an integrative approach to psychosocial and spiritual constructs. PRISM (Pictorial Representation of Illness and Self Measure) is a validated tool that measures the burden of psychosocial pain in patients with chronic cancer and other populations. Arranging sessions with a spiritual advisor, priest, or rabbi, meditation, or prayer are examples of interventions that play important roles in the approach to holistic palliation.

SUMMARY

Aggressively managing the symptoms of patients with critical life-limiting illness or terminal disease can improve the quality of life for the patient and their loved ones, regardless of how much time they have remaining. Palliative symptom management approaches disease in a holistic manner, addressing not only the physical aspect of symptoms but also the psychological, social, and spiritual dimensions of suffering for total symptom relief. Pain is the most common reason for critical care palliative consultation, and using the WHO pain ladder to systematically quantify, treat, and titrate pain management is effective. Treatment options include both pharmacologic and nonpharmacologic management. If treatments are burdensome and curative strategies are no longer in line with the patient's goals of care, transition to comfort care can be considered. The Hippocratic Oath summarizes our medical duty to do no harm and alleviate suffering by palliating, or "cloaking," the symptoms of illness and disease.

REFERENCES

1. The Advisory Board Company PEC. Realizing the full benefit of palliative care briefing. Palliative Care Executive Committee. 2013:9.

2. Delgado-Guay MO, Parsons HA, Li Z, et al. Symptom distress, interventions, and outcomes of intensive care unit cancer patients referred to a palliative care consult team. Cancer 2009;115(2):437–45.

3. Kross EK, Engelberg RA, Gries CJ, et al. ICU care associated with symptoms of depression and posttraumatic stress disorder among family members of patients who die in the ICU. Chest 2011;139(4):795–801.

4. Kelly AS, Deb P, Morrison RS. Hospice enrollment saves money for Medicare and improves care quality across a number of different lengths-of-stay. Health Aff (Millwood) 2013;32(3):552–61.

5. Luckett T, Phillips J, Agar M. Elements of effective palliative care models: a rapid review. BMC Health Serv Res 2014;14:136.

6. Gelfman LP, Meier DE, Morrison RS. Does palliative care improve quality? A survey of bereaved family members. J Pain Symptom Manage 2008;36(1):22–8.

7. Morrison RS. National palliative care research center; outcomes and quality standards. Orlando (FL): Center for Advanced Palliative Care; 2014.

8. Richardson J. A review of the reliability and validity of the Edmonton Symptom Assessment System. Curr Oncol 2009;16(1):55.

9. Vignaroli E, Pace EA, Willey J, et al. The Edmonton Symptom Assessment System as a screening tool for depression and anxiety. J Palliat Med 2006;9(2): 296–303.

10. Weinstein SM, Portenoy RK, Harrington SE. UNIPAC 3: assessing and treating pain. Glenview (IL): American Academy of Hospice and Palliative Medicine; 2012.

11. Vargas-Schaffer G. Is the WHO analgesic ladder still valid. Can Fam Physician 2010;56:514–7.

12. Takeda F. Pain theory and terminal illness: medical point of view. Assessment of Quality of Life and Cancer Treatment 1986;175–82.

13. Takeda F. Relief of cancer pain. Geneva (Switzerland): World Health Organization; 1986.

14. Rietjens JA, van Zuylen L, van Veluw H, et al. Palliative sedation in a specialized unit for acute palliative care in a cancer hospital: comparing patients dying with and without palliative sedation. J Pain Symptom Manage 2008;36:228–34.

15. McPherson ML. Demystifying opioid conversion calculations. a guide for effective dosing. Bethesda (MD): American Society of Health-System Pharmacists; 2010.

16. Goldstein NE, Morrison RS. Evidence-based practice of palliative care. Philadelphia: Elsevier Saunders; 2013.

17. Neu S, Kjellstrand CM. Stopping long-term dialysis. An empirical study of withdrawal of life-supporting treatment. N Engl J Med 1986;314:14–20.

18. Dean M. Opioids in renal failure and dialysis patients. J Pain Symptom Manage 2004;28:297–504.

19. Tucker R, Storey CP. Managing nonpain symptoms UNIPAC 4. Glenview (IL): AAHPM; 2012.

20. Gomutbutra P, O'Riordan DL, Pantilat SZ. Benzodiazepines and the management of dyspnea in palliative care patients. J Pain Symptom Manage 2012;45:374.

21. Glare P, Miller J, Nikolova T, et al. Treating nausea and vomiting in palliative care: a review. Clin Interv Aging 2011;6:243–59.

22. Meisner W, Schmidt U, Hartmann M, et al. Oral naloxone reverses opioid-associated constipation. Pain 2000;84:105–9.

23. Del Fabbro E, Hui D. Clinical outcomes and contributors to weight loss in a cancer cachexia clinic. J Palliat Med 2011;14(9):1004–8.

24. Peuckmann V, Elsner F, Krumm N. Pharmacologic treatments for fatigue associated with palliative care. Cochrane Database Syst Rev 2010;(11):CD006788.

25. Hisanaga T, Shinjo T, Morita T, et al. Multicenter prospective study on efficacy and safety of octreotide for inoperable malignant bowel obstruction. Jpn J Clin Oncol 2010;40:739–45.

26. Rosielle D, Marks S. Fast facts. End of Life/Palliative Education Resource Center. Center to Advanced Palliative Care; 2014. Available at: http://www.eperc.mcw.edu/EPERC/FastFactsandConcepts.

27. Rice AD, King R, Reed ED, et al. Manual physical therapy for non-surgical treatment of adhesion-related small bowel obstructions: two case reports. J Clin Med 2013;2:1–12.

Pediatric Palliative Care in the Intensive Care Unit

Kevin Madden, MD[a],*, Joanne Wolfe, MD[b], Christopher Collura, MD[c]

KEYWORDS

- Pediatrics • Palliative care • Intensive care • Intensive care units, neonatal
- Quality of life

KEY POINTS

- The patients cared for in Pediatric Palliative Care often have different diseases and trajectories of illness than those in the Adult Palliative Care setting.
- The chronicity of illness that afflicts children in Pediatric Palliative Care and the medical technology that has improved their lifespan and quality of life also make prognostication extremely difficult.
- The uncertainty of prognostication and the available medical technologies make both the neonatal intensive care unit (NICU) and the pediatric intensive care unit (PICU) locations where many children will receive Pediatric Palliative Care.
- Health care providers in the NICU and PICU should integrate fundamental Pediatric Palliative Care principles into their everyday practice.
- Specialized Pediatric Palliative Care providers should be consulted in complex life-threatening illnesses to provide concurrent strategies of supportive care in the acute phase of illness as well as over the course of the child's life.

INTRODUCTION

Pediatric palliative care (PPC) is an interdisciplinary specialty of which the ultimate goal is to ensure the best quality of life (QOL) for children with life-threatening illnesses by minimizing suffering from physical, psychological, emotional, or spiritual

The authors have nothing to disclose.
[a] Department of Palliative Care and Rehabilitation Medicine, University of Texas MD Anderson Cancer Center, 1515 Holcombe Boulevard, Unit 1414, Houston, TX 77030, USA; [b] Pediatric Palliative Care, Pediatric Palliative Care Service, Department of Psychosocial Oncology and Palliative Care, Children's Hospital Boston, Dana-Farber Cancer Institute, Harvard Medical School, DA2-012, 450 Brookline Avenue, Boston, MA 02215, USA; [c] Division of Neonatal Medicine, Department of Pediatric & Adolescent Medicine, Mayo Clinic College of Medicine, 200 First Street Southwest, Rochester, MN 55902, USA
* Corresponding author.
E-mail address: kmadden@mdanderson.org

Crit Care Nurs Clin N Am 27 (2015) 341–354
http://dx.doi.org/10.1016/j.cnc.2015.05.005
0899-5885/15/$ – see front matter © 2015 Elsevier Inc. All rights reserved.
ccnursing.theclinics.com

distress. "Interdisciplinary" is different than "multidisciplinary" in that each specialty retains its own identity, while simultaneously overlapping with each other in their guiding philosophy.[1] The construct of each PPC service is unique, depends on available resources, and includes a wide range of disciplines that reflect the underlying complex nature of delivering high-quality PPC. Team members can include a physician, nurse (registered or advanced practice), social worker, administrative assistant, chaplain, child life specialist, bereavement specialist, music therapist, art therapist, psychologist, massage therapist, pharmacist, physical therapist, occupational therapist, dietitian, and physician assistant.[2]

There are substantial differences between the fields of adult and pediatric palliative care. Although most adult palliative care patients have cancer, approximately 80% of children cared for by PPC teams have congenital, genetic, or neuromuscular disorders.[3] In addition, PPC is nascent; the first program was started in 1984, at St. Mary's Hospital for Children New York, and 2008 represented the peak in number of new hospital-based PPC programs established.[2]

EPIDEMIOLOGY AND DEMOGRAPHICS

The Centers for Disease Control and Prevention last released mortality data for the United States in 2013. In that year, approximately 43,000 children in the United States from birth to 19 years of age died and 10 times that number coped with a life-threatening condition. Most of those deaths (55%) were in infants less than 1 year of age.[4]

As evidenced from **Figs. 1** and **2**, many children die suddenly and unexpectedly, and so the provision of palliative care to them is questionable. It can be helpful, therefore, to examine causes of death due to a "complex chronic condition" (CCC). A CCC is defined as a medical condition that can be reasonably expected to last at least 12 months (unless death intervenes) and that involves either several different organ systems or one organ system severely enough to require specialty pediatric care

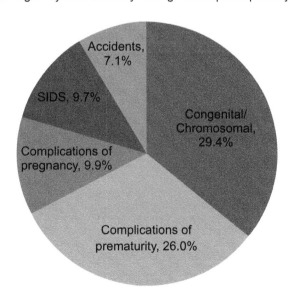

Fig. 1. Five leading causes of infant death (0–1 years of age). (*Data from* Centers for Disease and Control Prevention NCfIPaC. Leading causes of death reports, national and regional, 1999–2013. 2013. Available at: http://webappa.cdc.gov/sasweb/ncipc/leadcaus10_us.html. Accessed February 1, 2015.)

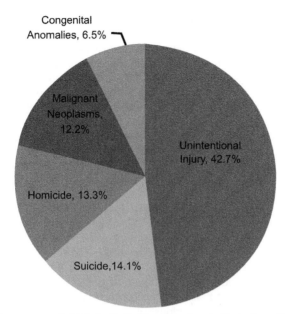

Fig. 2. Five leading causes of child death (1–19 years of age). (*Data from* Centers for Disease and Control Prevention NCfIPaC. Leading causes of death reports, national and regional, 1999–2013. 2013. Available at: http://webappa.cdc.gov/sasweb/ncipc/leadcaus10_us.html. Accessed February 1, 2015.)

and probably some period of hospitalization in a tertiary center.[5] A study looking at deaths in children from 1989 to 2003 concluded that approximately 22% of deaths occurred in children with a CCC, and of those children, the underlying CCC leading to death was fairly evenly distributed (**Fig. 3**).[6]

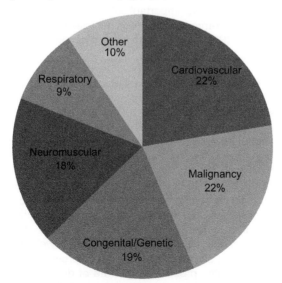

Fig. 3. Categories of disease that will lead to death in patients with a CCC. (*Data from* Feudtner C, Feinstein JA, Satchell M, et al. Shifting place of death among children with complex chronic conditions in the United States, 1989–2003. JAMA 2007;297(24):2725–32.)

The tremendous advancement of medical interventions and technology has transformed the world of Pediatrics. Illnesses that were once uniformly lethal within the first few days to months of life are now being successfully managed by novel surgical procedures, other therapeutic interventions, and the widespread availability of technology such as home ventilators. Children with CCCs are living longer than ever before and enjoy a QOL that was almost unimaginable 20 years ago. These complex interventions, however, mean that when these children do get ill, they are often directly admitted to an intensive care unit (ICU) that has the knowledge and expertise to manage their extraordinary care needs. The necessity of ICU clinicians to hold a primary responsibility to integrate PPC concepts into the care of their patients is tantamount, while subspecialty or dedicated PPC care providers should become involved in more complex situations and are responsible for research, innovation, and advocacy.

Although in the past 15 years there has been a shift to more deaths occurring at home,[6,7] the vast majority of children will die in hospitals. A consistent finding within the United States and abroad is that, for the most part, children who die in the hospital will almost invariably die in either a neonatal intensive care unit (NICU) or a pediatric intensive care unit (PICU), with estimated ranges of 80% to 91%.[8–13] Although it is not unusual for PPC providers to have years-long relationships with their patients due to the chronic nature of their underlying illness and the successful application of medical technology that allows seriously ill children to live longer, the large number of children who die in ICUs provides an opportunity to integrate philosophies and practices of PPC into these areas of care.

PALLIATIVE CARE IN THE NEONATAL INTENSIVE CARE UNIT

More than 23,000 babies die annually in the United States in their first year of life with the vast majority of these infants dying in the first 4 weeks of life.[14] The leading causes of infant death (see **Fig. 1**) also may portend severe morbidity and long-term disability for survivors. The NICU presents an important setting for integrated palliative care, not only for babies with acute life-threatening illness but also for those anticipated to have special health care needs (SHCN) and a high burden of complex pain and symptoms owing to severe neonatal illness.

The National Center for Health Statistics and Centers for Disease Control and Prevention use ICD-10 codes to quantify causes of infant deaths. These methods may dramatically underestimate the proportion of deaths related to complications of prematurity.[15] Babies born extremely preterm (less than 28 weeks' gestational age) have an overall in-hospital mortality rate of 273 per 1000 live births. These deaths are commonly related to severe complications of prematurity including lung disease, infection, necrotizing enterocolitis, or central nervous system injury. Approximately 40% of the time, death occurs within the first 12 hours of life.[16]

Neonates born at the threshold of viability and those with conditions predicting a high-risk of death or complications may trigger end-of-life decision-making. The American Academy of Pediatrics (AAP) offers guidance for providers for withholding resuscitation and discontinuing life-sustaining medical treatment (LSMT). Population-based data considering gestational age, birth weight, antenatal steroid administration, gender, and singleton pregnancy aid providers in predicting which extremely premature neonates present a high rate of death or potential long-term disability in survivors.[17,18] For these neonates, resuscitation is not indicated if the physician feels that there is no possibility for survival. If the clinical scenario presents less certainty, but outcomes including long-term neurodevelopmental impairment are considered potentially grave, parents' voices are central regarding the initiation of resuscitation.[19,20] For infants who undergo a trial of resuscitation, ongoing assessment and clear communication with parents are necessary as prognostic information becomes clinically available to best inform decision-making in the ICU.[21]

Most deaths in the NICU involve decisions to withhold resuscitative efforts at birth or discontinue LSMT.[22] The AAP directs compassionate comfort care for critically ill neonates for whom resuscitation or intensive care is not provided.[19,21] Practices in end-of-life care in the NICU have been shown to be variable and inconsistent.[23,24] This trend emphasizes the opportunities for enhanced palliative care skills in the care of neonates and potential partnership with PPC. Neonatologists express positive experiences with formal palliative care consultation,[25] but rates of neonates receiving formal PPC is low.[26] This relationship should be strengthened to allow benefits of consistent supportive care to exist in the critical environment of the NICU.

Former extremely preterm neonates experiencing morbidity in the NICU present an important population to consider concurrent methods of symptom-management, decision-making support, and coordination of care given their high rates of special health care needs (SHCN) (**Fig. 4**).

Congenital malformations and chromosomal abnormalities account for a leading cause of infant death; however, research indicates that deaths in babies with severe aneuploidy such as trisomy 13 and 18 may be overestimated by providers.[27,28] These infants receive significant medical and surgical interventions, often well into childhood.[29] PPC should play an integral role in the supportive and concurrent care for

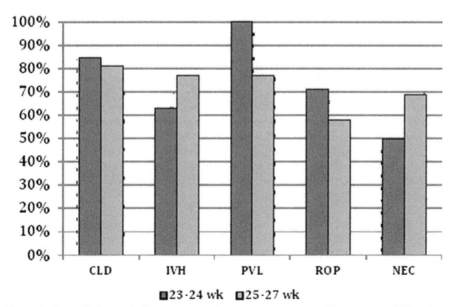

Fig. 4. SHCN at discharge in former extremely preterm neonates with severe morbidity. CLD, chronic lung disease; IVH, severe intraventricular hemorrhage; NEC, necrotizing enterocolitis; PVL, periventricular leukomalacia; ROP, retinopathy of prematurity. SHCN is defined as the need for home oxygen or monitors, medications, tube feeds, tracheostomy/mechanical ventilation, or ventriculoperitoneal shunt. (*Data from* Stephens BE, Tucker R, Vohr BR. Special health care needs of infants born at the limits of viability. Pediatrics 2010;125(6):1152–8.)

these children and families given the life-threatening nature of their illness, ongoing complex medical needs, and critical decision-making necessary to their care.

Children with life-threatening illness receiving palliative care are less likely to die in the ICU.[26] Formal consultation with PPC may improve this trend for neonates as well. PPC can provide coordinated expertise in facilitating discontinuation of LSMT in inpatient and outpatient settings outside of the NICU, optimizing a meaningful experience for parents.

A strategy for concurrent supportive care for children with CCCs is a core component of the PPC clinical relationship. Most children receiving PPC are alive for at least 1 year following consultation.[3]

PALLIATIVE CARE IN THE PEDIATRIC INTENSIVE CARE UNIT

With the explosion of available and easily transportable medical technology that allows children with chronic illnesses to reside outside of the hospital, it is not surprising that these technologically dependent children will often be admitted to a PICU when they become ill. Approximately 63% of children who die in the PICU had a chronic or pre-existing diagnosis, 15% had a gastrostomy tube, and 7% were dependent on mechanical ventilation, either through BiPAP (biphasic positive airway pressure) or a home ventilator.[30] There has not been extensive literature documenting the manner of death of children in the PICU, but it is estimated that 70% of children die by the discontinuation of LSMT, such as mechanical ventilation, cardiovascular support with vasopressors or extracorporeal membrane oxygenation, or renal dialysis; 16% were declared brain dead, and 14% had unsuccessful attempts at cardiopulmonary resuscitation.[30]

How to approach such delicate topics and the timing of advance care planning (ACP) discussions is a growing interest in Pediatrics. Most clinicians think that the optimal time for having such discussions is at time of diagnosis or in a period of medical stability, yet the reality is 71% of these same clinicians report that ACP happens too late, often when a child is acutely ill or near death.[31] Most clinicians (72%) admit that "not knowing the right thing to say" is "sometimes" or "often/always" a barrier to starting ACP discussions. Somewhat paradoxically, clinicians also report that the top 3 barriers to conducting ACP are (1) unrealistic parent expectations, (2) differences between clinician and parent/parent understanding of prognosis, and (3) lack of parent readiness to have the discussion. Nevertheless, less than 1% of clinicians think it is the parents' responsibility to initiate these discussions.[31] The outcome of clinicians thinking it is their responsibility to engage in ACP discussions but simultaneously not initiating them because of perceived barriers that reside primarily with parents is a communication "stalemate" whereby no conversation occurs and the child often suffers unnecessarily.

Seriously ill children nearing the end of life and their parents often have needs and desires that are unique and distinct from the adult population.[32] When considering the discontinuation of LSMT, parents' highest priorities are QOL, including the improvement of their child's pain.[33] Priorities of parents to improve the quality of care at the end of life in the PICU also include the following[34]:

1. Honest and complete information
2. Ready access to staff
3. Quality communication and care coordination
4. Provision of emotional expression and support by staff
5. Recognition of the importance of the parent-child relationship
6. Allowance and understanding of their personal faith

The communication gaps that exist and the issues identified above by parents represent a perfect opportunity for integrating the expertise and underlying philosophic principles of PPC providers with the highly technical knowledge and experience of PICU providers to collaboratively minimize the suffering of children nearing the end of life.

It is important to note, however, that the provision of PPC to children in the PICU should not be limited only to children nearing the end of life. The goals of all children and their families need to be elicited, and doing so can often have a profound impact on the child's journey. In Great Britain, children referred to PPC at discharge from the PICU were more likely to die in their home or hospice than children not referred to PPC services.[35]

COMMUNICATION

A recent meta-summary of qualitative analyses of patient and family needs in PPC highlighted the importance of advanced skills in communication.[36] The necessity of advanced skills in communication seems to be exceptionally true in the ICU, which can have negative effects on parents, who may experience a marginalized role in protecting their child.[37,38] Key domains such as support of the family unit, communication with the child and family about treatment goals and plans, and shared decision-making (SDM) have been underscored as essential to quality family-centered care in intensive care.[39]

Adult and pediatric providers in the ICU dominate interactions with families and relegate psychosocial concerns that may inform value-based preferences.[40–42] Parents of children who died in the ICU have identified multiple areas of needed attention in provider communication, including the following[43]:

- Physician availability and attentiveness
- Honesty and comprehensiveness of information
- Affect with which information was provided
- Withholding of information
- Contradictory information
- Physicians' body language

Pediatric staff members recognize inexperience in communication at end of life as well as transitions in palliative care.[44] Training in advanced communication can lessen dissatisfaction and may improve distress in the ICU.[45]

Critical decision-making for children with life-threatening illness should be rooted in a SDM model.

In addition to the principles described in **Table 1**, PPC providers should use advanced skills in communication to help families participate in value-based decision-making. Equally important in this process is the role of the child's primary medical team in making recommendations that align with a family's goals of care. The SDM asks the provider to take this active role in decision-making. This responsibility has advanced beyond the traditional informed model that simply tasked the physician to describe to the family all treatment or nontreatment options with their benefits and risks.[47]

REFRACTORY SYMPTOMS AT THE END OF LIFE

The treatment of symptoms commonly seen in PPC patients is not significantly different than in adults; with a few exceptions, the medications used are generally

Table 1 Ethical pediatric shared decision-making model	
Principle	**Description**
Family-centered	• Prioritize parental role in decision-making • Acknowledge parental values may diverge from providers[46]
Collaborative	• Provider not family holds independent decisional responsibility • All stakeholders decide together[47]
Value-driven	• Care tailored to racial, ethnic, sociocultural beliefs[48]
Truthful	• Provider duty to consistently deliver comprehensive, transparent, unbiased medical information[48]

Data from Refs.[46–48]

the same, although the dosages are obviously different. The treatment of symptoms is covered elsewhere in this issue (see article by Kittelson and colleagues).

Nevertheless, because most children with complex chronic medical conditions will die in the hospital, and not in the home or in hospice like adults, one can reasonably conclude then that PPC practitioners will often be in the position of caring for children who are at high risk for developing symptoms at the end of life that are difficult to treat with common interventions. Such symptoms are termed "refractory" and are defined as follows[49]:

1. Intensive efforts short of sedation fail to provide relief;
2. Additional invasive or noninvasive treatments incapable of providing relief;
3. Additional therapies associated with excessive or unacceptable morbidity or unlikely to provide relief within a reasonable time frame.

The treatment of refractory symptoms is through palliative sedation therapy (PST), an ethical[50] practice that uses specific medications to relieve intolerable suffering by reducing consciousness. Examples of such refractory symptoms include pain, delirium, and dyspnea.

The medical literature is sparse in regards to pediatric PST, and most guidelines and research come from the adult literature. Classes of medications commonly used in pediatric PST include opioids, benzodiazepines, antipsychotics, and barbiturates. Newer medications such as propofol (Diprivan) and dexmedetomidine (Precedex) are slowly gaining traction,[51–54] with the benefit of almost instantaneous onset of action, thus making them easily titratable to use the minimum dose needed to alleviate the specific refractory symptom.

There frequently is concern among family members and health care providers that PST may shorten the life,[55–57] but use of PST has been demonstrated not to hasten death.[58–60] Furthermore, it is crucial to highlight that PST is distinct from euthanasia because of the following:

1. It has the intent to provide symptom relief
2. It is a proportionate intervention
3. The death of the patient is not the intended goal

Although ethically acceptable, PST places an enormous burden on health care professionals and family members.[56,57,61] Therefore, PST should always occur in the context of clear, open communication with all staff members, including nursing, pharmacy, and physicians as well as the patient (if developmentally appropriate) and family members.

ETHICAL CONSIDERATIONS

PPC providers should be aware of unique ethical considerations in the care of children given the challenging nature of navigating childhood death.

Quality of Life

Pediatric decision-making regarding the limitation of potentially life-prolonging invasive interventions may lend itself to a family-driven assessment of the child's QOL. Such judgments can often lead to moral distress if there is disagreement between parents and providers in how the underlying illness impacts the child's life. Most people hold that some degree of neurologic function is necessary to espouse a minimal threshold of QOL.[62] Lantos and Meadow[63] argue that QOL should be carefully described in 4 subcomponents:

1. Anticipated cognitive or cerebral function
2. Anticipated physical disabilities
3. Pain and suffering associated with the illness
4. Burdens of future treatment

Research has demonstrated that parents are more likely than physicians and nurses to favor intensive treatment despite the high likelihood of significant associated underlying neurocognitive or psychomotor impairments.[64] In studies of adolescents with and parents of children with illness-related neurologic impairment, providers seem to overestimate how disability negatively impacts QOL.[65,66] In SDM, health care professionals should recognize personal value judgments may differ greatly than parents' in the qualitative assessment of a child's life and discretion should be used in communicating definitive neuroprognosis or anticipated QOL.

There may be rare instances that parents request limitations of LSMT that clearly run counter to providers' considerations of the child's best interest. In these instances, consultation with the hospital ethics committee may help determine potential conflicts and whether child protective mechanisms are indicated.[46]

Pediatric Assent

Family-centered decision-making for older children and adolescents should incorporate the voice of the patient as well as the parents.[67] Assent refers to a child's participation in decision-making and describes an empowering process[68] of developmental assessment of the child's decisional capacity; this includes his or her ability to understand relevant information, appreciate short- and long-term consequences, and express rational reasoning, including consistent risk-benefit considerations free from peer influence.[69] If an adolescent is assessed to have such capacity, providers should not only solicit assent in treatment decisions but also be willing to weigh these decisions seriously.[67]

Withholding Medically Provided Nutrition/Hydration

Withdrawing or forgoing medically provided nutrition and hydration (MPNH) remains controversial[70,71] despite statements from the American Medical Association[72] and AAP[73] that this treatment is not always indicated. Pediatric providers should acknowledge the sociocultural importance of providing food and liquids to newborns and children and never withhold feeds from patients able to safely orally eat or suck. However, for children unable to orally eat, the provision of nutrition and hydration supplied by enteral feeding tubes, pumps, and surgical procedures and requiring special formulas represents medical intervention.[74]

As in adults,[75] children with MPNH can suffer adverse complications, including fluid overload, electrolyte and nutritional imbalance, pain, and infection. Certain clinical situations may present ethically permissible decisions to withhold or withdraw MPNH in a child. These situations can include when a child permanently lacks awareness such as in a persistent vegetative state, or when MPNH clearly prolongs the dying process and presents additional sources of pain and suffering, such as in terminal illnesses like severe gastrointestinal malformations in infants.[74] Ethics consultation is encouraged in these circumstances given the uncommon nature of these events in children.

Duty to Care

Caring for a child with life-threatening illness imparts a duty of family-centered nonabandonment. Obligations of supportive care extend to a child's family members given the interconnectedness of the child's best interest with the well-being of the family as a whole. Nonabandonment should be forged through active presence in critical moments of a child's illness and through the child's death with parent and sibling bereavement.[76]

SPIRITUAL CARE

Parents report that faith and spirituality play an essential role in critical decision-making, coping with, and understanding their child's life-threatening illness.[34] Recent research demonstrates that parents with a spiritual focus might experience positive rather than negative emotions.[77] Parents of children who died in the PICU describe intense spiritual needs, including maintaining presence with their child, memory making, prayers, rituals, and connection with others.[78] Pediatric providers may miss opportunities to address spirituality and religion despite its importance.[79]

Chaplain integration into pediatric palliative interdisciplinary care teams is highly variable. Providers identify the meaningful value of chaplaincy in addressing spiritual suffering, enhancing communication, and attending to individualized rituals.[80] This integral aspect of care for families and children experiencing serious illness should be prioritized in order to optimize holistic family-centered care.

SUMMARY

PPC is a relatively young field, and so its integration into more established areas of hospitals is continuously evolving. The underlying fundamental principles of PPC are supportive of the child and family, with communication grounded in the SDM model and whose ultimate goal is to minimize the suffering of children and their families in all parts of their trajectory of illness, not just at the end of life. As most children will die in either a NICU or a PICU, it is paramount that PPC providers develop a collaborative relationship with their colleagues in the NICU and PICU so collectively they can provide the best care for seriously ill children at all stages of their life.

REFERENCES

1. Wolfe J, Hinds PS, Sourkes BM. Textbook of interdisciplinary pediatric palliative care. Philadelphia: Elsevier/Saunders; 2011.
2. Feudtner C, Womer J, Augustin R, et al. Pediatric palliative care programs in children's hospitals: a cross-sectional national survey. Pediatrics 2013;132(6): 1063–70.
3. Feudtner C, Kang TI, Hexem KR, et al. Pediatric palliative care patients: a prospective multicenter cohort study. Pediatrics 2011;127(6):1094–101.

4. Centers for Disease Control and Prevention NCfIPaC. Leading causes of death reports, national and regional, 1999-2013. 2013. Available at: http://webappa.cdc.gov/sasweb/ncipc/leadcaus10_us.html. Accessed February 1, 2015.
5. Feudtner C, Christakis DA, Zimmerman FJ, et al. Characteristics of deaths occurring in children's hospitals: implications for supportive care services. Pediatrics 2002;109(5):887–93.
6. Feudtner C, Feinstein JA, Satchell M, et al. Shifting place of death among children with complex chronic conditions in the United States, 1989-2003. JAMA 2007; 297(24):2725–32.
7. Schmidt P, Otto M, Hechler T, et al. Did increased availability of pediatric palliative care lead to improved palliative care outcomes in children with cancer? J Palliat Med 2013;16(9):1034–9.
8. Lantos JD, Berger AC, Zucker AR. Do-not-resuscitate orders in a children's hospital. Crit Care Med 1993;21(1):52–5.
9. Carter BS, Howenstein M, Gilmer MJ, et al. Circumstances surrounding the deaths of hospitalized children: opportunities for pediatric palliative care. Pediatrics 2004;114(3):e361–6.
10. Ashby MA, Kosky RJ, Laver HT, et al. An enquiry into death and dying at the Adelaide Children's Hospital: a useful model? Med J Aust 1991;154(3):165–70.
11. van der Wal ME, Renfurm LN, van Vught AJ, et al. Circumstances of dying in hospitalized children. Eur J Pediatr 1999;158(7):560–5.
12. McCallum DE, Byrne P, Bruera E. How children die in hospital. J Pain Symptom Manage 2000;20(6):417–23.
13. Ramnarayan P, Craig F, Petros A, et al. Characteristics of deaths occurring in hospitalised children: changing trends. J Med Ethics 2007;33(5):255–60.
14. Hamilton BE, Hoyert DL, Martin JA, et al. Annual summary of vital statistics: 2010-2011. Pediatrics 2013;131(3):548–58.
15. Callaghan WM, MacDorman MF, Rasmussen SA, et al. The contribution of preterm birth to infant mortality rates in the United States. Pediatrics 2006;118(4):1566–73.
16. Patel RM, Kandefer S, Walsh MC, et al. Causes and timing of death in extremely premature infants from 2000 through 2011. N Engl J Med 2015;372(4):331–40.
17. Tyson JE, Parikh NA, Langer J, et al. Intensive care for extreme prematurity–moving beyond gestational age. N Engl J Med 2008;358(16):1672–81.
18. Stoll BJ, Hansen NI, Bell EF, et al. Neonatal outcomes of extremely preterm infants from the NICHD Neonatal Research Network. Pediatrics 2010;126(3):443–56.
19. Batton DG, Committee on Fetus and Newborn. Clinical report–antenatal counseling regarding resuscitation at an extremely low gestational age. Pediatrics 2009;124(1):422–7.
20. Kattwinkel J, Perlman JM, Aziz K, et al. Neonatal resuscitation: 2010 American Heart Association Guidelines for Cardiopulmonary Resuscitation and Emergency Cardiovascular Care. Pediatrics 2010;126(5):e1400–13.
21. American Academy of Pediatrics Committee on Fetus and Newborn, Bell EF. Noninitiation or withdrawal of intensive care for high-risk newborns. Pediatrics 2007;119(2):401–3.
22. Barton L, Hodgman JE. The contribution of withholding or withdrawing care to newborn mortality. Pediatrics 2005;116(6):1487–91.
23. Cortezzo DE, Sanders MR, Brownell EA, et al. End-of-life care in the neonatal intensive care unit: experiences of staff and parents. Am J Perinatol 2014. [Epub ahead of print].
24. Janvier A, Meadow W, Leuthner SR, et al. Whom are we comforting? An analysis of comfort medications delivered to dying neonates. J Pediatr 2011;159(2):206–10.

25. Cortezzo DE, Sanders MR, Brownell E, et al. Neonatologists' perspectives of palliative and end-of-life care in neonatal intensive care units. J Perinatol 2013;33(9): 731–5.
26. Keele L, Keenan HT, Sheetz J, et al. Differences in characteristics of dying children who receive and do not receive palliative care. Pediatrics 2013;132(1):72–8.
27. Wilkinson DJ, Fitzsimons JJ, Dargaville PA, et al. Death in the neonatal intensive care unit: changing patterns of end of life care over two decades. Arch Dis Child Fetal Neonatal Ed 2006;91(4):F268–71.
28. Rasmussen SA, Wong LY, Yang Q, et al. Population-based analyses of mortality in trisomy 13 and trisomy 18. Pediatrics 2003;111(4 Pt 1):777–84.
29. Nelson KE, Hexem KR, Feudtner C. Inpatient hospital care of children with trisomy 13 and trisomy 18 in the United States. Pediatrics 2012;129(5):869–76.
30. Burns JP, Sellers DE, Meyer EC, et al. Epidemiology of death in the PICU at five U.S. teaching hospitals*. Crit Care Med 2014;42(9):2101–8.
31. Durall A, Zurakowski D, Wolfe J. Barriers to conducting advance care discussions for children with life-threatening conditions. Pediatrics 2012;129(4):e975–82.
32. Goldman A. ABC of palliative care. Special problems of children. BMJ 1998; 316(7124):49–52.
33. Meyer EC, Burns JP, Griffith JL, et al. Parental perspectives on end-of-life care in the pediatric intensive care unit. Crit Care Med 2002;30(1):226–31.
34. Meyer EC, Ritholz MD, Burns JP, et al. Improving the quality of end-of-life care in the pediatric intensive care unit: parents' priorities and recommendations. Pediatrics 2006;117(3):649–57.
35. Fraser LK, Miller M, Draper ES, et al. Place of death and palliative care following discharge from paediatric intensive care units. Arch Dis Child 2011;96(12): 1195–8.
36. Stevenson M, Achille M, Lugasi T. Pediatric palliative care in Canada and the United States: a qualitative metasummary of the needs of patients and families. J Palliat Med 2013;16(5):566–77.
37. Meyer EC, Snelling LK, Myren-Manbeck LK. Pediatric intensive care: the parents' experience. AACN Clin Issues 1998;9(1):64–74.
38. Miles MS, Funk SG, Carlson J. Parental stressor scale: neonatal intensive care unit. Nurse Res 1993;42(3):148–52.
39. Truog RD, Meyer EC, Burns JP. Toward interventions to improve end-of-life care in the pediatric intensive care unit. Crit Care Med 2006;34(11 Suppl):S373–9.
40. Selph RB, Shiang J, Engelberg R, et al. Empathy and life support decisions in intensive care units. J Gen Intern Med 2008;23(9):1311–7.
41. Clarke-Pounder JP, Boss RD, Roter DL, et al. Communication intervention in the neonatal intensive care unit: can it backfire? J Palliat Med 2015;18(2):157–61.
42. de Vos MA, Bos AP, Plotz FB, et al. Talking with parents about end-of-life decisions for their children. Pediatrics 2015;135(2):e465–76.
43. Meert KL, Eggly S, Pollack M, et al. Parents' perspectives on physician-parent communication near the time of a child's death in the pediatric intensive care unit. Pediatr Crit Care Med 2008;9(1):2–7.
44. Contro NA, Larson J, Scofield S, et al. Hospital staff and family perspectives regarding quality of pediatric palliative care. Pediatrics 2004;114(5):1248–52.
45. Truog RD, Campbell ML, Curtis JR, et al. Recommendations for end-of-life care in the intensive care unit: a consensus statement by the American College [corrected] of Critical Care Medicine. Crit Care Med 2008;36(3):953–63.
46. Ethics and the care of critically ill infants and children. American Academy of Pediatrics Committee on Bioethics. Pediatrics 1996;98(1):149–52.

47. Charles C, Whelan T, Gafni A. What do we mean by partnership in making decisions about treatment? BMJ 1999;319(7212):780–2.

48. Committee On Hospital Care, Institute For Patient, Family-Centered Care. Patient- and family-centered care and the pediatrician's role. Pediatrics 2012;129(2): 394–404.

49. Cherny NI, Portenoy RK. Sedation in the management of refractory symptoms: guidelines for evaluation and treatment. J Palliat Care 1994;10(2):31–8.

50. Burt RA. The Supreme Court speaks–not assisted suicide but a constitutional right to palliative care. N Engl J Med 1997;337(17):1234–6.

51. Anghelescu DL, Hamilton H, Faughnan LG, et al. Pediatric palliative sedation therapy with propofol: recommendations based on experience in children with terminal cancer. J Palliat Med 2012;15(10):1082–90.

52. de Graeff A, Dean M. Palliative sedation therapy in the last weeks of life: a literature review and recommendations for standards. J Palliat Med 2007;10(1):67–85.

53. McWilliams K, Keeley PW, Waterhouse ET. Propofol for terminal sedation in palliative care: a systematic review. J Palliat Med 2010;13(1):73–6.

54. Riker RR, Shehabi Y, Bokesch PM, et al. Dexmedetomidine vs midazolam for sedation of critically ill patients: a randomized trial. JAMA 2009;301(5):489–99.

55. Morita T, Ikenaga M, Adachi I, et al. Family experience with palliative sedation therapy for terminally ill cancer patients. J Pain Symptom Manage 2004;28(6): 557–65.

56. Morita T, Akechi T, Sugawara Y, et al. Practices and attitudes of Japanese oncologists and palliative care physicians concerning terminal sedation: a nationwide survey. J Clin Oncol 2002;20(3):758–64.

57. Rietjens JA, Hauser J, van der Heide A, et al. Having a difficult time leaving: experiences and attitudes of nurses with palliative sedation. Palliat Med 2007;21(7): 643–9.

58. Maltoni M, Pittureri C, Scarpi E, et al. Palliative sedation therapy does not hasten death: results from a prospective multicenter study. Ann Oncol 2009;20(7): 1163–9.

59. Chiu TY, Hu WY, Lue BH, et al. Sedation for refractory symptoms of terminal cancer patients in Taiwan. J Pain Symptom Manage 2001;21(6):467–72.

60. Morita T, Tsunoda J, Inoue S, et al. Effects of high dose opioids and sedatives on survival in terminally ill cancer patients. J Pain Symptom Manage 2001;21(4): 282–9.

61. Morita T, Miyashita M, Kimura R, et al. Emotional burden of nurses in palliative sedation therapy. Palliat Med 2004;18(6):550–7.

62. Rhoden NK. Treatment dilemmas for imperiled newborns: why quality of life counts. S C Law Rev 1985;58(6):1283–347.

63. Lantos JDM, Meadow WL. Neonatal bioethics. Baltimore (MD): Johns Hopkins University Press; 2006.

64. Streiner DL, Saigal S, Burrows E, et al. Attitudes of parents and health care professionals toward active treatment of extremely premature infants. Pediatrics 2001;108(1):152–7.

65. Saigal S, Lambert M, Russ C, et al. Self-esteem of adolescents who were born prematurely. Pediatrics 2002;109(3):429–33.

66. Feingold E, Sheir-Neiss G, Melnychuk J, et al. HRQL and severity of brain ultrasound findings in a cohort of adolescents who were born preterm. J Adolesc Health 2002;31(3):234–9.

67. Bartholome WG. Informed consent, parental permission, and assent in pediatric practice. Pediatrics 1995;96(5 Pt 1):981–2.

68. King NM, Cross AW. Children as decision makers: guidelines for pediatricians. J Pediatr 1989;115(1):10–6.
69. Frader JE, Flanagan E. Minors as decision makers. In: Adam MD, Diekema DS, Mercurio MR, editors. Bieothics resident curriculum: case-based teaching guide. Elk Grove Village (IL): American Academy of Pediatrics; 2011. p. 32–7.
70. Solomon MZ, Sellers DE, Heller KS, et al. New and lingering controversies in pediatric end-of-life care. Pediatrics 2005;116(4):872–83.
71. Feltman DM, Du H, Leuthner SR. Survey of neonatologists' attitudes toward limiting life-sustaining treatments in the neonatal intensive care unit. J Perinatol 2012;32(11):886–92.
72. Decisions near the end of life. Council on Ethical and Judicial Affairs, American Medical Association. JAMA 1992;267(16):2229–33.
73. American Academy of Pediatrics Committee on Bioethics: guidelines on foregoing life-sustaining medical treatment. Pediatrics 1994;93(3):532–6.
74. Diekema DS, Botkin JR, Committee on Bioethics. Clinical report–forgoing medically provided nutrition and hydration in children. Pediatrics 2009;124(2):813–22.
75. Winter SM. Terminal nutrition: framing the debate for the withdrawal of nutritional support in terminally ill patients. Am J Med 2000;109(9):723–6.
76. Jones BL, Contro N, Koch KD. The duty of the physician to care for the family in pediatric palliative care: context, communication, and caring. Pediatrics 2014; 133(Suppl 1):S8–15.
77. Feudtner C, Walter JK, Faerber JA, et al. Good-parent beliefs of parents of seriously ill children. JAMA Pediatr 2015;169(1):39–47.
78. Meert KL, Thurston CS, Briller SH. The spiritual needs of parents at the time of their child's death in the pediatric intensive care unit and during bereavement: a qualitative study. Pediatr Crit Care Med 2005;6(4):420–7.
79. King SD, Dimmers MA, Langer S, et al. Doctors' attentiveness to the spirituality/ religion of their patients in pediatric and oncology settings in the Northwest USA. J Health Care Chaplain 2013;19(4):140–64.
80. Fitchett G, Lyndes KA, Cadge W, et al. The role of professional chaplains on pediatric palliative care teams: perspectives from physicians and chaplains. J Palliat Med 2011;14(6):704–7.

Palliative Care in the Emergency Department

Laurence M. Solberg, MD*, Jacobo Hincapie-Echeverri, MD

KEYWORDS

- Palliative care • Emergency department • Delirium • Pain control • Quality of life

KEY POINTS

- Palliative care (PC) initiated in the emergency department (ED) is an innovative idea that is now incorporated more frequently across health care settings.
- The ED typically treats immediate symptom and pain relief and historically does not initiate PC.
- Different models of PC in the ED can deliver services in consultation with the PC team or with PC champions in the ED.
- Barriers to the implementation of PC in the ED include a lack of research on this topic, which inhibits informed policy making.

BACKGROUND

The emergency department (ED) is a fast-paced environment in which patients seek immediate relief of pain and other distressing symptoms. Emergency physicians are trained to provide care that focuses on disease-directed treatment of acute illnesses.[1] In an effort to stabilize patients and preserve life, emergent procedures and treatments for medical conditions are often provided. Despite this, many patients with chronic or end-stage diseases seek treatment and assistance for their conditions in the ED each year. Thus, the ED is frequently the point of entry into the health care system for acute episodes of illness in a patient's life.

In 2004, more than 90% of Medicare beneficiaries were hospitalized in the year before death; more than 50% of those with serious illness in the United States died in the hospital.[2] Surveys of healthy adults suggest that most would like to die at home; however, most Americans still die in the hospital. Care in the ED is traditionally aggressive in nature; conversely, it is also episodic. Therefore, this environment is not

The authors have nothing to disclose.
Division of Geriatric Medicine, Department of Aging and Geriatric Research, University of Florida College of Medicine, 2004 Mowry Road, Mailbox 112610, Gainesville, FL 32610, USA
* Corresponding author.
E-mail address: LMSolberg@ufl.edu

Crit Care Nurs Clin N Am 27 (2015) 355–368
http://dx.doi.org/10.1016/j.cnc.2015.05.008
0899-5885/15/$ – see front matter Published by Elsevier Inc.
ccnursing.theclinics.com

usually considered a place to initiate palliative care (PC). The opposing nature of emergency care has placed it at odds with the traditional PC culture.[3]

The ED sees a variety of patient populations, and the decisions within the ED greatly impact the patients' hospital stay and goals of care. As health care resources become more strained and inpatient PC has gained more recognition, literature has emerged calling for the presence of PC in the ED. EDs are seeing older and more complex patients who are in need of PC for relief of exacerbations of a chronic condition. Older patients or patients with end-stage cancer may not desire aggressive treatments in the ED but may seek palliation of symptoms that are more in agreement with their goals of care and the patients' interpretation of quality of life. Chronic diseases are now the leading causes of death (**Table 1**).[4] These diseases have a high prevalence of physical, psychosocial, spiritual, and financial suffering associated with complex illness.[1] Other patients seeking care in the ED may be patients with cancer who are either receiving or have received chemotherapy and are having side effects of the treatment for which outpatient management has failed. Residents of long-term care facilities (nursing homes, rehabilitation facilities) can be medically complex and require the ED physician to have a discussion on the goals of care or review an advanced directive with patients and/or the families. These roles are ones in which the ED physician may not be well versed.

When discussing PC it is important to note that there is a distinction between hospice care and PC. PC is focused on communication, comfort, and quality of life and can be used at the same time as life-prolonging treatments. This approach to care is conducive to the treatment of chronic serious diseases and conditions whereby the goal is to decrease suffering and in doing so achieve the best quality of life possible for the patients.[5] Hospice care typically begins as restorative or curative care is finishing and end of life is near; however, it continues after the death of the patients in the form of bereavement support for the family.

PRESENTING TO THE EMERGENCY DEPARTMENT FOR PALLIATIVE CARE

The absence or presence of PC in the ED largely depends on the extent of a PC program at the individual hospital. A greater number of patients receiving PC in the

Table 1
Chronic diseases in the top 10 causes of death in the United States

Rank	Disease	Deaths Per Year	Percentage Total Deaths (%)
1	Heart disease	596,577	23.71
2	Cancer (malignant neoplasms)	576,691	22.92
3	Chronic lower respiratory disease	142,943	5.68
4	Stroke (cerebrovascular diseases)	128,932	5.12
5	Accidents (unintentional injuries)	126,438	5.02
6	Alzheimer disease	84,974	3.37
7	Diabetes (diabetes mellitus)	73,831	2.93
8	Influenza and pneumonia	53,826	2.13
9	Kidney disease (nephritis, nephrotic syndrome, and nephrosis)	45,591	1.81
10	Suicide (intentional self-harm)	39,518	1.57

Data from Nichols H. What are the top 10 leading causes of death in the US? Medical News Today. Available at: http://www.medicalnewstoday.com/articles/282929.php#top_10_leading_causes_of_death. Accessed March 16, 2015.

community and hospital will likely lead to an increase in the utilization of both ED and hospital PC resources.[6] Although evidence shows that patients and families prefer PC to be at home, most note that they will go to the ED if symptoms are uncontrolled.[7] Barbera, Taylor, and Dudgeon[8] noted that palliative patients often find visiting the ED "distressing, exhausting and disruptive."[8] This finding shows that ED physicians will need to have PC education and training to serve these patients. Use of the ED for PC in the United States has been noted in studies (**Table 2**).

GAPS IN PALLIATIVE CARE IN THE EMERGENCY DEPARTMENT

There are gaps in services and education regarding PC in the ED. In order to better serve patients who are seeking PC in the ED, there has been a growth in the PC fellowship

Table 2
Studies of incidence of patients with PC needs presenting to the ED in the United States

Author	Study Aims	Country	Sample Size	Study Findings
Earle et al,[9] 2004	To evaluate trends in the aggressiveness of cancer care over 4 y	United States	28,277	From the years 1993–1996, there was an increase from 7.2% to 9.2% ($P \leq .001$) in the use of the ED by patients with these cancers.
Grudzen et al,[10] 2010	To explore the palliative care needs of older adults in the ED	United States	50	PC needs of older adults in the ED were not limited to just physical symptoms; patients also experienced mental distress, financial difficulties, caregiving needs that were unmet, and difficulty in accessing care.
Glajchen et al,[11] 2011	To assess PC needs among elderly patients presenting to the ED	United States	144	144 patients with life-limiting conditions presented to the ED over 8 mo of the study.
Warren et al,[12] 2011	To compare end-of-life care between the United States (Medicare) and Ontario, Canada for patients with NSCLC	United States, Canada	Medicare (13,533), Ontario (8100)	End-of-life care for patients with NSCLC was different between Medicare and Ontario. It was found that there were fewer Medicare patients that used the ED as well as hospitalizations in comparison with those in Ontario.

Abbreviation: NSCLS, non–small cell lung cancer.
Data from Refs.[9–12]

programs nationwide. In 2006 the American Board of Medical Specialties approved the creation of hospice and palliative medicine as a subspecialty. At that time less than 70 fellowship programs existed. Now there are 108 fellowship programs in the United States that are recognized by the American Council of Graduate Medical Education.[13] Despite these programs, there is a shortage of PC physicians to care for these patients. The National Priorities Partnership identified PC as one of 6 priority areas that impact and improve key patient-centered quality and utilization outcomes.[14] To demonstrate the support and encouragement of PC in the ED, the American Board of Emergency Medicine officially sponsored hospice and palliative medicine as a subspecialty.[1]

Additionally, education on PC issues in the ED is lacking.[2] In response to the increasing number of patients entering the ED for PC, PC competencies have been created throughout residency training, which includes geriatrics and PC.[15] Furthermore, emergency medicine provider curricula in PC, the "Education in Palliative and End-of-Life Care for Emergency Medicine," has emerged.[16] Topics include quick steps for performing a rapid PC assessment in the ED; formulation of trajectories and prognoses based on the clinical judgment and validated indexes[17]; the care of hospice patients, patients who have cancer, and patients who experience chronic pain; and family witnessed resuscitation. Techniques for teaching PC to other emergency practitioners are also taught.[16] These programs assist ED physicians to become more comfortable with the subject of PC.

DIFFERENT MODELS OF PALLIATIVE CARE IN THE EMERGENCY DEPARTMENT

To address the growing needs of patients and the gaps in care that occur, different models of PC exist to assist the provider in the ED. Some hospitals use the integrative model of care, in which ED providers implement primary PC interventions with each patient. Still others have PC champions in the ED who have partnered with hospice providers in their area.[18] Most EDs use the consultative method with an external, hospital-based PC team. This interdisciplinary PC team can assess and assist in the treatment of symptoms, support decision making, initiate spiritual well-being, help align treatments to support patient and family goals, and also start contacting resources for practical aid for patients and their family caregivers. Regardless of the model used, PC in the ED has shown to be effective and cost-efficient.

The consultation of a PC team is the most common model in the ED. At Virginia Commonwealth University Medical Center, there was a significantly greater financial impact for those admitted and consulted for PC in the ED.[19] In the Columbus, Ohio Mount Carmel Health System, there were 3 hospitals that had PC teams consulting in the ED. These teams worked with the ED and developed screening tools specifically for their cohort of patients. These teams also attended ED staff meetings and rounded in the ED. This partnership of PC and emergency medicine in the Mount Carmel Health System demonstrated that EDs were the source of 9.2% of all admissions to the PC units and of 66.7% of all direct admissions to the PC unit from the ED.[20]

Another model for PC in the ED used an integrative approach, with the use of PC champions. Because PC is a subspecialty of emergency medicine, there are ED physicians who are board certified in palliative medicine. Physicians certified in both disciplines can serve as champions for PC in the ED. A pilot program was started by one such physician in Scripps Mercy Hospital in San Diego, California, which initiated PC consults on patients while in the ED and not admitted yet to the hospital. The results showed approximately 37% of those patients consulted were able to be admitted to hospice agencies, suggesting it is feasible for ED patients to be transferred to hospice care without admission to the hospital.[21]

EMERGENCY DEPARTMENT PARTNERSHIPS WITH HOSPICE

As noted previously, the partnership with hospice agencies can benefit patients seen in the ED, especially for end-of-life issues. One such partnership is demonstrated at University of Florida Health Hospital in Jacksonville, Florida where a close partnership with community hospice agencies and 2 PC nurses in the ED allowed for early identification of patients whose symptoms can be managed as outpatients and were eligible for hospice benefits. Often times, care is sought in the ED to provide effective palliation of symptoms for patients with life-altering or life-limiting illness. Preliminary data from this project showed that this program allowed more patients to be discharged home with hospice care from the ED, avoiding a hospital admission.[22] The partnership with community hospice agencies is important for the transition of care to occur in a timely and effective manner.

PALLIATIVE CARE SYMPTOM MANAGEMENT IN THE EMERGENCY DEPARTMENT

Patients present to the ED for a variety of symptoms and concerns, some are related to the disease process itself and others are a result of treatments for or progression of the disease. The ED can provide symptom management and referrals to assist patients with meeting their goals of care. Kotajima and colleagues[23] described patients with lung cancer who presented to the ED with both cancer-related and cancer-unrelated issues. The cancer-unrelated issues were symptoms of chronic diseases incidentally occurring in patients with cancer. Dyspnea, fever, and pain were the most common complaints in this cohort of patients, comprising 62% of cancer-related issues in patients and 72% of cancer-unrelated issues in patients. Although similar numbers of patients with lung cancer presented to the ED with cancer-related issues (70 patients) and cancer-unrelated issues (73 patients), there were less complaints of fever in the cancer-related cohort[7] versus the cancer-unrelated group.[22] This difference was the only statistically significant difference in the groups.[23] The patients with cancer-related issues showed a shorter survival time: 61 days versus 406 days (**Fig. 1**).

SYMPTOM MANAGEMENT IN THE EMERGENCY DEPARTMENT: PAIN

The most common PC symptoms that present to the ED include pain (45.1%),[24,25] anorexia (34.0%), constipation (32.0%), weakness (32.0%), and dyspnea (31.0%).[25,26] Pain continues to be one of the most prevalent and distressing symptoms in PC, especially at the end of life, with 64% of patients reporting pain.[26] Pain in patients with cancer may be from the cancer, from physiologic conditions related to the cancer, from treatment of the cancer, or caused by another condition, chronic or acute, that is not related to the cancer.

Palliative pain management has not been adequately studied in the ED. Pain management in the PC setting (outside of the ED) describes long-term dosing as a more effective manner to control the pain.[27] The highest rate of severe pain is seen in patients with end-stage cancer.[28] In another study, it is noted that no specific code exists for pain-related crisis, so they combined all the diagnoses involving pain in various body sites (ie, abdomen, chest, back, or limb) and found that these accounted for 9.4% of visits made during the final 6 months and 5.1% of visits made during the final 2 weeks of life.[8]

Pain management in the ED should follow a stepwise approach, as outlined in the principles of the World Health Organization Pain Relief Ladder.[29] *The first step* is to use nonopioid medications, such as nonsteroidal antiinflammatories. If the pain is not relieved, then care progresses to *the second step*, which uses a weak opioid for

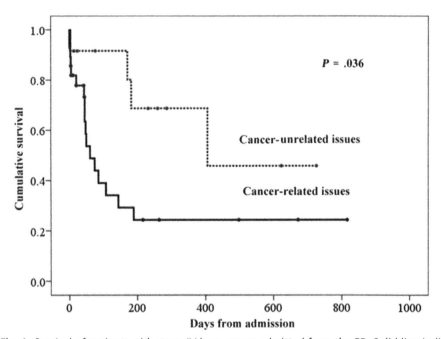

Fig. 1. Survival of patients with stage IV lung cancer admitted from the ED. Solid line indicates survival curve of patients admitted for cancer-related issues; the dotted line indicates survival curve of patients admitted for cancer-unrelated issues. The patients admitted for cancer-related reasons exhibited a significantly shorter median survival time compared with those admitted for cancer-unrelated issues (61 vs 406 days, respectively; $P<.05$). (*From* Kotajima F, Kobayashi K, Sakaguchi H, et al. Lung cancer patients frequently visit the emergency room for cancer related and-unrelated issues. Mol Clin Oncol 2014;2(2):325; with permission.)

mild to moderate pain, which is added to the nonopioid medication. If this combination does not relieve the pain, then *the third step* is used, which substitutes the weaker opioid for a strong opioid for moderate to severe pain. If a medication stops being effective along the process, do not change to a medication of the same step; use a stronger medication to achieve pain relief.[29] Management with opioids is the treatment of choice; however, it is often underutilized because of fears of causing respiratory depression.[30] A detailed pain management discussion can be found within this journal by Kittelson and colleagues.

SYMPTOM MANAGEMENT IN THE EMERGENCY DEPARTMENT: DELIRIUM

Another common symptom that brings PC patients to the ED is delirium. The data from the literature demonstrate a prevalence of delirium between 13% and 88% and an incidence between 3% and 45%.[31] Delirium is a clinical diagnosis based on standard criteria.[32] The diagnostic criteria of delirium from the *Diagnostic Statistical Manual of Mental Disorders*, Fifth Edition (*DSM-5*) shows the standards in terms of diagnosis based on the best available evidence and expert consensus at the time of publication. The *DSM-5* diagnostic criteria for delirium are[33]

1. There is a disturbance in attention (ie, reduced ability to direct, focus, sustain, and shift attention) and awareness (reduced orientation to the environment).

2. The disturbance develops over a short period of time (usually hours to a few days), represents a change from baseline attention and awareness, and tends to fluctuate in severity during the course of a day.
3. There is an additional disturbance in cognition (eg, memory deficit, disorientation, language, visuospatial ability or perception).
4. The disturbances in criteria 1 and 2 are not better explained by another preexisting, established, or evolving neurocognitive disorder and do not occur in the context of a severely reduced level of arousal, such as coma.
5. There is evidence from the history, physical examination, or laboratory findings that the disturbance is a direct physiologic consequence of another medical condition, substance intoxication or withdrawal (ie, because of a drug of abuse or to a medication), or exposure to a toxin or is a result of multiple causes.[33]

Studies suggest that delirium is reversible in almost half of the cases within PC, whereas, in terminal disease, it is typically irreversible or coined *terminal delirium*. Terminal delirium is the result of advanced disease and organ failure and less from infectious or medication-related causes.[34,35] This type of delirium is different from intensive-care-unit (ICU) delirium, which is related more to the severity of acute illness, with metabolic and medication-induced causes.[36] Delirium in the PC setting is grossly underdiagnosed[37,38] partly because of the lack of routine screening but also because of the waxing and waning nature of the condition. Detection in the ED is also difficult because testing for delirium in this setting is not standardized or a usual focus of care. The current literature shows that there are approximately 16% to 18% of older adults who are delirious on entry to the ED.[39] Hypoactive delirium has a various prevalence, 68% to 86 % in certain studies and 20% in others,[37] being the most frequently missed form of delirium because of the frequent overlap of symptoms with depression[40]; it has also been associated with early mortality.[41] Similarly, hyperactive delirium can masquerade as anxiety, mania, or akathisia.[42] Screening for delirium in PC patients is difficult, but there are several screening tools that have shown to be effective **(Table 3)**.[42]

The primary goal for treating delirium is to reverse the underlying cause after it is identified. There is an increase of elderly patients visiting the ED, most of those with multiple comorbidities and medications that are used for symptom relief. One common cause, polypharmacy, should be considered. The cessation of medications that can cause delirium and the rotation of opioid medications is an initial intervention. Another common cause in this population is dehydration and the associated hyponatremia or hypercalcemia, which should be treated.[43]

Other common causes for delirium in this population are

- Infections secondary to an already decreased immune system (urinary tract infections, aspiration pneumonia, *Clostridium difficile*, pressure ulcer infections, cellulitis)
- Pain
- Nutritional deficiencies (thiamine, folic acid, B_{12})
- Withdrawal of medications (patients may be prescribed benzodiazepines or opioids)
- Other acute metabolic changes (acidosis, hypoglycemia/hyperglycemia, hypokalemia/hyperkalemia)
- Toxicities secondary to possible decreased liver metabolism or renal excretion (chemotherapy, anticonvulsants, antiarrhythmics, anxiolytics, analgesics, antidepressants, illicit drugs, biological therapy, steroids, anticholinergic drugs, psychoactive drugs)

Table 3
Characteristics of delirium tools used in PC populations

Category	Scale	Dimensions	Items	Score	Administration Time (min)	Characteristics
Delirium screening	CAM	9 Operationalized criteria based on *DSM-III-R*, classified as 4 features	9	Observational	5[a]	• Required for diagnosis: features 1 (acute 2 (inattention) + either feature 3 (disorganized thinking) or 4 (altered level of consciousness)
	Nu-DESC	4 items from the CRS + psychomotor retardation	5	0–10 Cutoff: ≥2	1	• 3-Point scale: 0–2 • Observational scale • Higher score = positive delirium
	SQiD	Third-party perception of patients' confusion	1	Yes/no	—	• Simple single question • Perception of family member/friend
Delirium severity	DRS-R-98	13 Severity items (including 5 cognitive domains), 3 diagnostic items	16	0–39 (Severity) 0–46 (total) Cutoff: 15.25 (severity) Cutoff: 17.75 (diagnostic)	20–30	• Items rated from zero (normal) to 3 (severely impaired) • Symptoms rated over 24 h • Higher score = increased severity • 13-Item severity section can be scored separately from 3-item diagnostic section • Total scale can be scored initially to enhance differential diagnosis
	MDAS	Based on *DSM-IV, DSM-III,* and *ICD-9* criteria: arousal and LOC cognitive functioning psychomotor activity	10	0–30 Diagnostic cutoff: 7–13	10	• 4-Point scale: 0–3 • Higher score = increased severity
Neuropsychological assessment of delirium for research purposes	CTD	Orientation, attention, memory, vigilance, and comprehension	—	0–30 Cutoff: <19	20	• Lower score = lower cognitive function

Abbreviations: CAM, Confusion Assessment Method; CRS, Cognation Rating Scale; CTD, Cognitive Test for Delirium; DRS-R-98, Delirium Rating Scale-Revised; *DSM-III-R, Diagnostic and Statistical Manual of Mental Disorders* (Third Edition Revised); *ICD-9, International Classification of Diseases, Ninth Revision;* LOC, level of consciousness; MDAS, Memorial Delirium Assessment Scale; Nu-DESC, Nursing Delirium Screening Scale; SQiD, Single Question in Delirium.

a For experienced users.

From Leonard MM, Nekolaichuk C, Meagher DJ, et al. Practical assessment of delirium in palliative care. J Pain Symptom Manage 2014;48(2):176–90; with permission.

Table 4
Antipsychotics for the management of delirium

Drug[a–c]	Mechanism of Action	Dosing Per Day/Route of Administration	Clinical Characteristics and Pearls	Side Effects and Precautions
Typical APs				
Haloperidol (Haldol)	DA	0.5–10.0 PO, IV, IM, SC	First choice in delirium (recommended by guidelines) RCTs available Antiemetic properties	Monitor QTc Extrapyramidal effects common
Chlorpromazine (Thorazine)	DA	12.5–200 mg IV, IM, SC	Anxiolytic and sedative effects RCTs available	Monitor QTc, sedation, hypotension
Methotrimeprazine (Nozinan)	—	PR 6.25–12.25 PO, IV, SC	Analgesic, antiemetic, and sedating effects	Anticholinergic side effects common (constipation, dry mouth, blurred vision, tachycardia): NB in patients in opioid treatment and poly-drug therapy
Atypical APs				
Olanzapine, (Zyprexa, Zyprexa Zydis, Symbyax, Zyprexa Intramuscular, Zyprexa Relprevv)	MARTA	2.5–20.0 PO, IM, SC	Sedating effects Appetite stimulant and antiemetic properties RCT available (vs risperidone)	Monitor QTc Anticholinergic side effects (constipation, dry mouth)
Quetiapine, (Seroquel)	MARTA	25–300 PO	Sedative effects Hypotension RCT available (vs haloperidol; vs amisulpride)	Monitor QTc Sedation
Risperidone, (Risperdal, Risperdal Consta, Risperdal M-Tab)	SDA	0.25–6.0 mg PO	Less side effects vs typical APs if in low doses (otherwise as haloperidol) RCT available (vs olanzapine)	Monitor QTc Possible extrapyramidal effects
Ziprasidone, (Geodon)	SDA	40–160 PO, IM	Sedating profile No RCT	Monitor QTc and EKG Few research in delirium

(continued on next page)

Table 4
(continued)

Drug[a-c]	Mechanism of Action	Dosing Per Day/Route of Administration	Clinical Characteristics and Pearls	Side Effects and Precautions
Other atypical APs				
Aripiprazole (Abilify, Abilify Maintena, Abilify Discmelt)	DPA	5–20 PO, IM	Less side effects of typical APs Data on efficacy in hypoactive delirium	Monitor QTc Agitation, possible extrapyramidal symptoms
Perospirone (generic)	SDA	5–15 PO	Effective in 86.8% of cases Effect within several days No RCT	Reported low incidence of side effects (fatigue, sleepiness, akathisia, hypotension)
Amisulpride (generic)	DA (D2 and D3); GA	150 PO	Effective in delirium, RCT available (vs quetiapine)	Few side effects

Abbreviations: AP, antipsychotic; DA, dopamine antagonist; DPA, dopamine partial agonist; EKG, electrocardiogram; GA, γ-hydroxybutyrate agonist; IM, intramuscular; IV, intravenous; MARTA, multi-acting receptor-targeted antipsychotics; NB, note well; PR, per rectum; RCT, randomized controlled trial; SC, subcutaneous; SDA, serotonin–dopamine antagonist.

[a] Recommendations in oncology and PC settings.[34]

[b] Neurological symptoms (eg, extrapyramidal symptoms, including dystonias, akathisia, and Parkinsonian symptoms; reduction of seizure threshold): monitor at baseline and daily.

[c] Cardiologic symptoms: blood pressure and pulse at baseline and at least daily (closer or continuous monitoring for at-risk or medically unstable patients); electrocardiogram at baseline and with every AP dose increase or daily if high doses of AP are used (closer attention to patients with underlying unstable cardiac disease, electrolyte disturbances, or on other QTc prolonging medications for the increased risk of torsades des pointes).

Adapted from Grassi L, Caraceni A, Mitchell AJ, et al. Management of delirium in palliative care: a review. Curr Psychiatry Rep 2015;17(3):1–9; with permission.

- Central nervous system insults (stroke, meningitis, intracranial bleeding, metastatic disease)
- Endocrinopathies (hypothyroidism/hyperthyroidism, hypoglycemia/hyperglycemia, adrenal insufficiency)
- Cardiac/pulmonary causes (heart failure, shock, pulmonary embolism, malignancy, vasculitis), hypoxia
- Constipation or urinary retention
- Noise, excess visual stimuli, sleep disturbance
- Restraints while in the ED and/or an unfamiliar environment

Therefore, a careful history, clinical examination, and ordering of patient-specific laboratory tests are mandatory for the evaluation and treatment of delirium. Laboratory tests to consider include (1) complete blood cell count, (2) electrolytes, renal and liver function tests, (3) analysis of urine, (4) arterial blood gas, (5) chest radiograph, (6) electrocardiogram, and (7) appropriate cultures. Additionally, a careful evaluation of the medication administered and the possible interactions and cognitive side effects should be evaluated.[44]

Pharmacologic and nonpharmacologic interventions also may be used to treat the delirium. The details of these treatments are outside the scope of this article. The antipsychotics are commonly used to treat delirium in clinical settings and in PC. Several meta-analyses have shown that antipsychotics are effective treatments for delirium[45,46] (Table 4).

Research in PC has demonstrated that multicomponent nonpharmacologic interventions, such as orientation, mobility, and reducing sleep disturbances, are effective in reducing the precipitation of delirium.[32,47] Also shown to be valuable are educational and behavioral interventions for patients and spouses because high levels of distress have been seen by nursing staff caring for delirious patients at the end of life.[48]

SUMMARY

The benefits of PC are well supported within the literature. The data from Morrison and colleagues[2] demonstrate associated reductions in hospital costs and a significant decrease in length of stay. Inpatients who were discharged to home who had received PC services had significant reductions in laboratory and ICU charges resulting in decreased costs compared with usual-care patients, with an adjusted net savings of $1696 in direct costs per admission ($P = .004$) and $279 in direct costs per day ($P = .001$). The PC patients who died in the hospital had an adjusted net savings of $4908 in direct costs per admission ($P = .003$) and $374 in direct costs per day ($P = .001$), which included significant reductions in pharmacy, laboratory, and ICU costs when compared with usual-care patients.[49]

Currently, there are little research and evidence on the use of PC in the ED. However, one may infer patient satisfaction: other outcomes will improve and costs will be reduced, as it has in the inpatient setting. The systematic integration of PC into the ED is slowly occurring, as it is a recognized subspecialty of emergency medicine. Offering PC in the ED will benefit patients, families, and hospitals.[1] The lack of data regarding PC in the ED is a potential barrier to evidence-based policymaking; nonetheless, patients and their families will benefit from palliative services in the ED. Further study is needed to better describe the anticipated benefits of PC in the ED.

REFERENCES

1. Grudzen CR, Stone SC, Morrison RS. The palliative care model for emergency department patients with advanced illness. J Palliat Med 2011;14(8):945-50.

2. Morrison RS, Maroney-Galin C, Kralovec PD, et al. The growth of palliative care programs in United States hospitals. J Palliat Med 2005;8(6):1127–34.

3. Grudzen CR, Richardson LD, Hopper SS, et al. Does palliative care have a future in the emergency department? Discussions with attending emergency physicians. J Pain Symptom Manage 2012;43(1):1–9.

4. Available at: http://www.medicalnewstoday.com/articles/282929.php#top_10_leading_causes_of_death. Accessed March 16, 2015.

5. Guidelines for quality palliative care. Clin Prac. 2009. Available at: www.nationalconsensusproject.org. Accessed March 8, 2015.

6. Wallace EM, Cooney MC, Walsh J, et al. Why do palliative care patients present to the emergency department? Avoidable or unavoidable? Am J Hosp Palliat Care 2013;30(3):253–6.

7. Robinson J, Gott M, Ingleton C. Patient and family experiences of palliative care in hospital: what do we know? An integrative review. Palliat Med 2014;28(1):18–33.

8. Barbera L, Taylor C, Dudgeon D. Why do patients with cancer visit the emergency department near the end of life? Can Med Assoc J 2010;182(6):563–8.

9. Earle CC, Neville BA, Landrum MB, et al. Trends in the aggressiveness of cancer care near the end of life. J Clin Oncol 2004;22(2):315–21.

10. Grudzen CR, Richardson LD, Morrison M, et al. Palliative care needs of seriously ill, older adults presenting to the emergency department. Acad Emerg Med 2010;17(11):1253–7.

11. Glajchen M, Lawson R, Homel P, et al. A rapid two-stage screening protocol for palliative care in the emergency department: a quality improvement initiative. J Pain Symptom Manage 2011;42(5):657–62.

12. Warren JL, Barbera L, Bremner KE, et al. End-of-life care for lung cancer patients in the United States and Ontario. J Natl Cancer Inst 2011;103(11):853–62.

13. Available at: http://www.acgme.org/acgmeweb/. Accessed March 8, 2015.

14. Meier DE. Increased access to palliative care and hospice services: opportunities to improve value in health care. Milbank Q 2011;89(3):343–80.

15. Hogan TM, Losman ED, Carpenter CR, et al. Development of geriatric competencies for emergency medicine residents using an expert consensus process. Acad Emerg Med 2010;17(3):316–24.

16. EPEC-EM. Available at: www.epec.net/epec_em.php. Accessed March 8, 2015.

17. Available at: www.eprognosis.com. Accessed March 9, 2015.

18. O'Mahony S, Blank A, Simpson J, et al. Preliminary report of a palliative care and case management project in an emergency department for chronically ill elderly patients. J Urban Health 2008;85(3):443–51.

19. Meier DE, Beresford L. Palliative care in inpatient units. J Palliat Med 2006;9(6):1244–9.

20. Meier DE, Beresford L. Fast response is key to partnering with the emergency department. J Palliat Med 2007;10(3):641–5.

21. Waugh DG. Palliative care project in the emergency department. J Palliat Med 2010;13(8):936.

22. Hendry H, McIntosh M, Borgman P, et al. Integrating hospice and palliative care services in the ED: effects on resident and faculty education and ED overcrowding. New Orleans (LA): Society of Academcy Emergency Medicine; 2009.

23. Kotajima F, Kobayashi K, Sakaguchi H, et al. Lung cancer patients frequently visit the emergency room for cancer-related and-unrelated issues. Mol Clin Oncol 2014;2(2):322–6.

24. Strassels SA, Blough DK, Hazlet TK, et al. Pain, demographics, and clinical characteristics in persons who received hospice care in the United States. J Pain Symptom Manage 2006;32(6):519–31.
25. Potter J, Hami F, Bryan T, et al. Symptoms in 400 patients referred to PC services: prevalence and patterns. Palliat Med 2003;17(4):310–4.
26. Steinhauser KE, Arnold RM, Olsen MK, et al. Comparing three life-limiting diseases: does diagnosis matter or is sick, sick? J Pain Symptom Manage 2011; 42(3):331–41.
27. Pereira J, Lawlor P, Vigano A, et al. Equianalgesic dose ratios for opioids: a critical review and proposals for long-term dosing. J Pain Symptom Manage 2001; 22(2):672–87.
28. Solano JP, Gomes B, Higginson IJ. A comparison of symptom prevalence in far advanced cancer, AIDS, heart disease, chronic obstructive pulmonary disease and renal disease. J Pain Symptom Manage 2006;31(1):58–69.
29. World Health Organization. Cancer pain relief: with a guide to opioid availability. Washington, DC: World Health Organization; 1996.
30. Romem A, Tom SE, Beauchene M, et al. Pain management at the end of life: a comparative study of cancer, dementia, and chronic obstructive pulmonary disease patients. Palliat Med 2015;29(5):464–9.
31. Caraceni A, Grassi L. Delirium: acute confusional states in palliative medicine. UK: Oxford University Press; 2011.
32. Inouye SK, Westendorp RG, Saczynski JS. Delirium in elderly people. Lancet 2014;383(9920):911–22.
33. American Psychiatric Association. Diagnostic and statistical manual of mental disorders (DSM). Washington, DC: American Psychiatric Association; 1994. p. 143–7.
34. Lawlor PG, Gagnon B, Mancini IL, et al. Occurrence, causes, and outcome of delirium in patients with advanced cancer: a prospective study. Arch Intern Med 2000;160(6):786–94.
35. Breitbart W, Strout D. Delirium in the terminally ill. Clin Geriatr Med 2000;16(2): 357–72.
36. Pun BT, Ely EW. The importance of diagnosing and managing ICU delirium. Chest 2007;132(2):624–36.
37. Rainsford S, Rosenberg JP, Bullen T. Delirium in advanced cancer: screening for the incidence on admission to an inpatient hospice unit. J Palliat Med 2014;17(9): 1045–8.
38. Fang CK, Chen HW, Liu SI, et al. Prevalence, detection and treatment of delirium in terminal cancer inpatients: a prospective survey. Jpn J Clin Oncol 2008;38(1): 56–63.
39. Sanon M, Baumlin KM, Kaplan SS, et al. Care and respect for elders in emergencies program: a preliminary report of a volunteer approach to enhance care in the emergency department. J Am Geriatr Soc 2014;62(2):365–70.
40. Leonard M, Spiller J, Keen J, et al. Symptoms of depression and delirium assessed serially in palliative-care inpatients. Psychosomatics 2009;50(5):506–14.
41. Meagher DJ, Leonard M, Donnelly S, et al. A longitudinal study of motor subtypes in delirium: relationship with other phenomenology, etiology, medication exposure and prognosis. J Psychosom Res 2011;71(6):395–403.
42. Leonard MM, Nekolaichuk C, Meagher DJ, et al. Practical assessment of delirium in palliative care. J Pain Symptom Manage 2014;48(2):176–90.
43. Caruso R, Grassi L, Nanni MG, et al. Psychopharmacology in psycho-oncology. Curr Psychiatry Rep 2013;15(9):1–10.

44. Caraceni A, Simonetti F. Palliating delirium in patients with cancer. Lancet Oncol 2009;10(2):164–72.

45. Grassi L, Caraceni A, Mitchell AJ, et al. Management of delirium in palliative care: a review. Curr Psychiatry Rep 2015;17(3):1–9.

46. Tahir TA. A review for usefulness of atypical antipsychotics and cholinesterase inhibitors in delirium. Pharmacopsychiatry 2012;45(4):163 [author reply: 164].

47. Maldonado JR. Pathoetiological model of delirium: a comprehensive understanding of the neurobiology of delirium and an evidence-based approach to prevention and treatment. Crit Care Clin 2008;24(4):789–856.

48. Breitbart W, Gibson C, Tremblay A. The delirium experience: delirium recall and delirium-related distress in hospitalized patients with cancer, their spouses/caregivers, and their nurses. Psychosomatics 2002;43(3):183–94.

49. Morrison RS, Penrod JD, Cassel JB, et al. Cost savings associated with US hospital PC consultation programs. Arch Intern Med 2008;168(16):1783–90.

Healing Environments
Integrative Medicine and Palliative Care in Acute Care Settings

Irene M. Estores, MD[a],*, Joyce Frye, DO, MBA, MSCE[b]

KEYWORDS

- Integrative medicine • Palliative care • Mind body medicine • Spirituality
- Essential oil therapy • Homeopathy • Biofield therapies • Massage

KEY POINTS

- Physical, mental, or emotional distress associated with a hospital admission remains difficult to treat with conventional therapies.
- An integrative approach to support patients during acute and critical illness improves safety, increases comfort, and enhances the innate healing response.
- Staff should be offered access to skills training to cultivate compassion and mindful practice to enhance both patient care and self-care.

INTRODUCTION
Integrative Medicine

Integrative medicine, as defined by the Academic Consortium for Integrative Medicine and Health, is the practice of medicine that reaffirms the importance of the relationship between practitioner and patient, focuses on the whole person, is informed by evidence, and makes use of all appropriate therapeutic approaches, health care professionals, and disciplines to achieve optimal health and healing. Complementary modalities such as acupuncture, massage, meditation, art therapy, music therapy, guided imagery, essential oil therapy, and biofield therapies, have been safely and effectively used in acute care settings to provide nondrug symptom management.[1–4] More important, it is an approach that addresses the physical environment, relationships, conversations, and behaviors, not only for patients but also for families and for health care professionals providing care in acute care settings, and truly integrates the mind, body, and spirit in the work of healing.

[a] Integrative Medicine Program, Division of General Internal Medicine, University of Florida College of Medicine, Gainesville, FL, USA; [b] Pharmacopeia Revision Committee, Homeopathic Pharmacopeia Convention of the United States, Baltimore, MD, USA
* Corresponding author.
E-mail address: Irene.estores@medicine.ufl.edu

Crit Care Nurs Clin N Am 27 (2015) 369–382
http://dx.doi.org/10.1016/j.cnc.2015.05.002
0899-5885/15/$ – see front matter © 2015 Elsevier Inc. All rights reserved.
ccnursing.theclinics.com

CURRENT PRACTICE GAPS IN ACUTE CARE

Conventional medicine is excellent at saving lives; however, it has little to offer to address the physical, mental, and emotional distress associated with life-threatening or life-limiting disease. For example, many patients experience some level of anxiety and pain during a hospital admission, whether it is from the medical or surgical condition that precipitated their admission, or with procedures used to treat these conditions. Additionally, patients and their families are left on their own to find processes to create meaning and to help them adjust to the altered circumstances of their lives in a manner that contributes to the positive, transformative, and resilient aspects of healing and psycho-spiritual growth.[5] Anxiety, nausea, and pain are symptoms that remain difficult to treat safely and adequately with conventional therapies, yet significantly affect quality of life.

The National Quality Forum is an organization that addresses both safety and quality in hospital care. In its *Safe Practices for Better Healthcare* 2009 Update, the National Quality Forum asked how the current health care system could better manage pain (improve quality) while simultaneously reducing side effects (improve safety). The report further stated, "There is strong evidence that integrative care can heal and improve basic conventional care by addressing the mind, body and spirit connection." The Joint Commission revised its pain management standards for 2015, recognizing that both pharmacologic and nonpharmacologic strategies have a role in the management of pain. The need and practice gap are increasingly being recognized. Adopting an integrative approach to palliative care in acute care settings can meet this need and fill this gap.

STRATEGIES FOR THE PHYSICAL ENVIRONMENT
Stimulus Modulation

Intensive care settings provide unremitting sensory stimulation. Excessive light and noise disrupt circadian rhythms, resulting in poor sleep quality and delirium.[6,7] The circadian rhythm secretion pattern of melatonin as measured by urine 6-sulfotoxymelatonin levels is disrupted in critically ill, septic patients.[8] Sleep pattern disruptions, in the form of predominant stage 1 sleep, less rapid eye movement (REM) and slow-wave sleep, rebound after REM deprivation, reduced total sleep time and sleep efficiency, frequent sleep stage transitions, and greater proportions of daytime sleep have also been reported.[8] Stimulus modulation practices to address sleep disruption include the use of eye masks, turning off artificial lights, and decreasing noise and movement. As a part of patient-centered care, standard hospital practices and incorporation of patient and family preferences should be reviewed to allow for improved sleep. These measures include adjusting feeding, laboratory and diagnostic testing, vital signs monitoring, and medication administration schedules by eliciting information from the patient and family members about particular practices that promote sleep, or the use of sleep objects.[9]

Reducing Health Care–Acquired Infections

Hospital-acquired infections, especially in intensive care units (ICUs), result in significant patient morbidity and mortality and drive costs.[10] A wide range of infection control measures, including patient isolation, hand and surface disinfection, changing practices in antibiotic prescribing and use of indwelling devices, and development of new antiinfective agents are being used to address this. Metals and essential oils with antiinfective properties are two complementary modalities that can potentially be added to this array.

The medicinal use of metals with biocidal properties is reported in the Edwin Smith papyrus (1500 BC) where copper salt was described as an astringent.[11] The Ayurvedic system of medicine, dating back to 5000 BC, likewise has a rich tradition of using heavy metals and minerals in refined compounded forms (gold, silver, copper, iron, tin, lead) as part of its pharmacopeia.[12]

Therapeutic applications of metals with inherent biocidal properties to decrease surface bioburden in current acute care settings are being studied. Examples include the following:

- Copper
  - Reduction in the rate of hospital-acquired infections and/or methicillin-resistant *Staphylococcus aureus* or vancomycin-resistant *Enterococcus* colonization in patients receiving care in ICU rooms with copper alloy surfaces than patients in standard ICU rooms[13]
- Silver
  - Historical use of silver nitrate also has a long history of medicinal use as a disinfectant.[11]
  - Broad-spectrum bioactivity of silver nanoparticles with effects on multiple classes of infectious pathogens as well as cancer.[14]
  - Use of a silver hydrogel urethral catheter to reduce symptomatic catheter-associated urinary tract infection[15]

Essential Oil Therapy

Additional strategies for reducing and treating hospital-acquired infections include the use of essential oils—the volatile organic constituents of plants. Commonly known as aromatherapy, the use of scent for creating a more pleasant environment as well as for disguising unpleasant odors goes back to time immemorial. The effects of aroma can be rapid, and sometimes just thinking about a smell can be as powerful as the actual smell itself.[16] Essential oils are thought to work at psychological, physiologic, and cellular levels beyond their aromatic effects.[17] Examples include the following:

- Essential oils mix (primarily eucalyptus) to treat malodorous necrotic ulcers in cancer patients significantly decreased odor, improved quality of life, and even promoted tissue healing.[18]
- Lavender for relaxation has a demonstrated physiologic effects in the brain.[19]
- Aromatherapy massage improved anxiety and depression in cancer patients for up to 2 weeks after the intervention.[20]
- Sweet marjoram for chronic, antibiotic-resistant, *Clostridium*–infected pressure ulcer responding to topical treatment with a 5% solution of sweet marjoram.[21]

Combinations may be more effective than single oils. In vitro studies demonstrate which combinations are active against various strains of multi–drug-resistant pathogens.[22] Combining essential oils with antibiotics can also produce synergistic effects that are more powerful than either treatment alone.[23,24] Similar to antibiotics, the choice of essential oils combination must be appropriate to the organism(s) being treated. Tea tree oil (*Melaleuca alternifolia*) in the form of a 5% body wash did not reduce methicillin-resistant *S aureus* compared with a Johnson's Baby Softwash in a group of critically ill patients.[25] However, in a separate study, tea tree oil was found to be more potent against gram-negative bacteria, and lemon oil was more effective against gram-positive organisms.[26] **Table 1** (taken from *Clinical Aromatherapy: Essential Oils in Healthcare*) gives examples of essential oils combinations along with sensitive pathogens and method of assessing efficacy.[21]

Table 1
Essential oils for resistant infections

Author, Year	Essential Oil	Pathogen	Method
Silva et al, 2013	Thyme oregano pennyroyal	*Pseudomonas aeruginosa, Enterococcus faecalis*	Agar diffusion
Duarte et al, 2012	*Coriandrum sativum*	*Acinetobacter baumannii*	Improved effectiveness of ciprofloxacin, gentamicin and tetracycline
Vegh et al, 2012	*Lavandula vera L intermedia L pyrenaica L stoechas*	*P aeruginosa*	Tube dilution containing 0.2% polysorbate 80
Hamoud et al, 2012	Peppermint Olbas	MRSA VRE	Kill time assay
Lysakowska et al, 2012	*Thymus vulgaris*	*Acinetobacter baumannii*	Agar diffusion
Tyagi et al, 2010	Lemongrass, *Mentha arvensis,* peppermint, *Eucalyptus globulus*	*P aeruginosa*	Vapor and liquid diffusion
Owlia, 2009	*Zataria multiflora Myrtle communis Eucalyptus camaldulensis*	*P aeruginosa*	Disk diffusion
Roller et al, 2009	*Lavandula angustifolia L latifolia L stoechas L luisieri*	MRSA	Direct contact
Doran et al, 2009	Lemongrass Geranium	MRSA VRE *A baumannii Clostridium difficile*	Diffused into air
Jazani et al, 2009	Fennel: *Foeniculum vulgare*	*A baumannii*	48 isolates from humans; disc diffusion
Hosseini et al, 2008	Cumin	MDR *P aeruginosa*	52 burn isolates from 2 hospitals
Chao et al, 2008	Lemongrass, lemon myrtle, mountain savory, cinnamon, melissa	MRSA	Disc diffusion
Dryden et al, 2004	Teatree	MRSA	Human study 224 patients
Opalchenova, 2003	Basil: *Ocimum basilicum*	MDR *P aeruginosa* MRSA MDR *E coli*	Kill time assay

Abbreviations: MDR, multidrug resistant; MRSA, methicillin-resistant *Streptococcus aureus*; VRE, vancomycin-resistant enterococcus.

From Buckle J. Clinical aromatherapy: essential oils in practice. 3rd edition. Philadelphia: Churchill Livingstone; 2014; with permission.

NONDRUG MODALITIES FOR SYMPTOM MANAGEMENT

Pain, agitation, and delirium are frequently observed in acute care settings[27] and pharmacologic symptom management relies heavily on opioids, benzodiazepines, and antipsychotics. Patients consequently experience other distressing symptoms, such as nausea and constipation secondary to use of these drugs.[28] Several nondrug modalities for symptom management can be integrated into current practice to improve care and decrease harms.

Acupuncture and Acupressure

Acupuncture is believed to work by regulating the flow of energy, called *qi*, traveling along energy channels in the body called *meridians*. In Traditional Chinese Medicine theory, any imbalance or stagnation of this flow results in disease. Needles, pressure, or heated herbs applied to specific acupuncture points along the body are used to restore this balanced flow. The debate continues on the efficacy of acupuncture as a therapeutic modality.[29] Nevertheless, in the 2007 National Health Interview Survey, 6.3% of the population, representing 14.01 million adults reported lifetime use, and 1.4% (ie, 3.14 million American adults) reported recent use of acupuncture.[30] However, its use is still limited in hospitals compared with ambulatory settings.[31] Examples include the following:

- Prevention of atrial fibrillation after coronary artery bypass graft surgery: Study protocol was acceptable to staff, patients, and family and was considered safe for these patients; however, the protocol was not feasible as designed and, therefore, the efficacy of acupuncture could not be determined.[32]
- Adjunct to pharmacologic therapy of postoperative pain after total hip and total knee replacement: Average short-term pain reduction using a self-reported numeric rating scale (1–10), assessed before and after acupuncture.[33]
- Electroacupuncture using a standard acupuncture protocol was more effective than sham acupuncture or no acupuncture and resulted in shorter time to defecation and decreased analgesic requirement after laparoscopic colorectal surgery.[34]

Acupressure typically uses only the practitioner's hands to restore the balance of qi in a noninvasive way that may be more readily employed in acute care. It can also be used in children or others who are afraid of needles. Small studies report reductions in pain, nausea, vomiting, and anxiety during labor and delivery and after surgery.[35–37]

Art Therapy

Art in the hospital setting can be an accessible place to begin the conversations necessary to provide tools for the management of mental and emotional health and to create a reflective self-care regimen. Creating meaning and connection for difficult life events through a nonverbal medium offers empowerment in situations that are overwhelming and serves to reframe negative ideas about illness or issues. In one study, women with cancer in a Mindfulness Based Art Therapy program had significant improvements in health-related quality of life.[38] Patients who had survived a myocardial infarction were asked to draw pictures of their heart at 3 and 6 month follow-up visits. Drawings of the heart that were larger in size correlated with significantly greater cardiac anxiety, more phone calls to health services, increased activity restriction, and slower return to work.[39]

A qualitative study conducted by Sonke and colleagues[40] on the impact of arts in medicine programming demonstrated positive effects on staff outcomes (job satisfaction, stress, unit culture) and patient outcomes on a short-term medical-surgical unit, and negative effects, with music being shown to be a distraction for staff.

Mind–Body Practices

Guided imagery, guided meditation, hypnosis, and other terms are similar methods for creating mental focus — in this case focusing on pleasant experiences and sensations rather than pain and anxiety (**Box 1**).

Massage

The use of touch for healing is as old as humankind. All cultures have used touch in healing. Most patients receiving massage in acute settings reported increased relaxation, a sense of well-being, and positive mood change, and attributed enhanced mobility, greater energy, increased participation in treatment, and faster recovery to massage therapy.[50] Massage can be combined readily with aromatherapy with the simple addition of essential oils to the massage oil or lotion. Companions and volunteers can also perform simple massage techniques, such as hand massage. Indeed, the intervention may be as therapeutic for the stressed caregiver, who is at a loss for words, as it is for the patient. Examples include the following:

- Reductions in self-reported distress for pain, physical discomfort, emotional discomfort, and fatigue in patients at a university hospital oncology unit after receiving massage, regardless of gender, age, ethnicity, or cancer type.[51]
- Immune preservation in children positive for human immunodeficiency virus infection.[52]
- Increase in the number of circulating lymphocytes and decrease in markers of inflammation as well as levels of arginine vasopressin was seen in a single session of Swedish massage performed on healthy volunteers.[53]

Box 1
Examples of mind–body practices

- Hypnosis
  - Self-hypnosis before surgery to reduce postoperative pain, nausea, analgesic requirements, and postoperative recovery time.[41]
  - Hypnotic language learned and used by nonhypnotist health care professionals increases patient comfort, and decreases costs during interventional and diagnostic procedures[42–44]
- Guided imagery
  - Use of a standard guided imagery message, such as a PlayAway, a packaged a single message MP3 unit, for patients before surgery to reduce anxiety and duration of stay.[45]
- Yoga
  - Patients with chronic obstructive pulmonary disease have been shown to have significant improvements in standard measures of respiratory function and quality of life after a 6-week yoga training program.[46]
  - Endurance, strength, balance, quality of life, and mood in patients with stable congestive heart failure all improved with yoga training.[47]
  - Faster healing of acute using yogic prana energy technique.[48]
  - Improvements in mood and decreases in anxiety and levels of GABA, similar to changes seen with antidepressants in subjects receiving yoga compared with walking.[49]

Data from Refs.[41–49]

- Increase in oxytocin and reductions in adrenocorticotrophic hormone, nitrous oxide, and β-endorphin after a 15-minute shoulder and neck massage in healthy persons compared with a rest group.[54]
- Decreased pain, anxiety, and tension in postoperative cardiac patients who received massage therapy had significantly decreased compared with a control group.[55]

Homeopathy

Homeopathy is the 200-year-old system of medicine founded by German physician Samuel Hahnemann.[56] Although less used in the United States, the World Health Organization indicates it is the second most used medicine worldwide.[57] In the United States, the manufacture and sale of homeopathic medicines is regulated by the Food and Drug Administration.[58] Highly dilute (potentized) forms of what would otherwise be toxic substances are used for their hormetic effect; that is, small doses stimulate whereas high doses inhibit.[59] Often disparaged owing to the high dilutions used, researchers now suggest that nanoparticles generated in the potentization process are responsible for the clinical effects.[60,61] Marzotto and associates investigated the gene expression of a human neurocyte cell line treated with increasing dilutions of *Gelsemium sempervirens* extract. With microarray hybridization, gene expression was seen to be affected in 56 genes, 2 of which (TAC4 and GALR2) may be of particular importance as they are involved in the psycho–neuro–immune–endocrine axis that relates emotional responses to hormone release and immune functions.[62]

Homeopathic medicines may be delivered by sublingual, topical, intravenous, rectal, or inhalation routes. Medicines are classically chosen individually to match the full spectrum of a patient's mental, emotional, and physical symptoms rather than solely on the basis of their condition. Examples include the following:

- Sepsis
  - In a randomized, controlled trial, patients in an ICU with systemic infections (sepsis) were 50% more likely to be alive at 6 months if treated with individual homeopathy compared with placebo.[63]
- Mechanical ventilation
  - In another study at the same ICU, patients with excess secretions on mechanical ventilation were able to be extubated and discharged from the ICU 3.5 days earlier when given a specific homeopathic medicine (potassium bichromate).[64]
- Abdominal surgery
  - In a metaanalysis combining the results of several smaller studies, homeopathic treatment shortened the time to first flatus after abdominal surgery.[65]
- Anxiety
  - Homeopathically prepared *Gelsimium sempervirens*, is commonly prescribed for anticipatory anxiety. Animal studies demonstrate reduction in anxiety behavior comparable with buspirone without the adverse effects on sedation or locomotion,[66,67] and a 30-day seizure prevention in a rat model of induced status epilepticus that resumed after cessation.[68]

Biofield Therapies

The National Center for Complementary and Integrative Health collectively includes modalities such as reiki, healing touch, therapeutic touch, pranic healing, qigong, distance healing, and laying of hands, as biofield therapies. The National Center for Complementary and Integrative Health defines biofields as "putative energy fields that have defied measurement to date by reproducible methods." The use of subtle energies for healing has likewise been in use for millennia, across cultures and spiritual traditions. The evidence for most of the perceived benefits of these modalities is anecdotal and has not been demonstrated in randomized, controlled trials or in recent best evidence synthesis.[69,70] However, in a study comparing 8 sessions of biofield therapy with mock healing and wait-list control for breast cancer–related fatigue, both biofield and mock healing significantly reduced fatigue, but only biofield therapy significantly decreased the cortisol slope.[71]

THERAPEUTIC MUSIC

Throughout history, music and sound have been used to alleviate physical, mental, and emotional pain. Shamans used medicine songs to promote healing, the Hindus used a specific pitch system known as ragas, and indigenous tribes used sweat lodges and 'singings' to promote healing."[72] Patients in a transplant unit receiving 15- to 35-minute sessions consisting of live, patient-preferred music and therapeutic social interaction demonstrated significant improvement in self-reported levels of anxiety, relaxation, pain, and nausea.[73]

SPIRITUAL SUPPORT

Life-limiting illness carries a high burden of suffering for the patient, their families, and health care professionals. Health care professionals work amid sickness and suffering, and become immersed in the struggles of suffering persons for meaning and spiritual direction. Although we are becoming a more religiously pluralistic and secularized society, spiritual practices and beliefs may still provide a way to improve coping and find meaning in the midst of this suffering. The task of providing spiritual support to patients in hospitals has typically been delegated to hospital chaplains and spiritual care providers. To truly provide holistic and compassionate care, spiritual care should be integrated into clinical care. Information on any cultural, religious, or spiritual beliefs or practices that influence a patient's health behaviors and decisions can be elicited.

Spirituality conveys numerous meanings, but if viewed broadly as a connection to what one holds as meaningful in life, it can be woven into patient interactions with more ease. Craigie[74] suggests inviting a conversation by asking questions such as, "What sustains you and keeps you going through hard times?" or "When have been some times when you have felt really alive?"

RELATIONSHIPS AND CONVERSATIONS
Mindful Use of Language

The body possesses an innate ability for self-healing and self-regulation. Its systems interact to maintain internal stability and homeostasis, despite internal fluctuations or external injury. All physical healing modalities—be they drug, surgery, or botanicals—aim to promote this self-healing process. The manner by which treatments are presented enhances their effect. The placebo effect is recognized as a real phenomenon and can be used to enhance the outcome of therapeutic interventions. One way to elicit the placebo effect is through the use of language. Kaptchuk and co-workers[75] demonstrated proof of this concept in a randomized trial involving patients with irritable bowel syndrome. Consider using a language of comfort and elicit patient and family preferences and practices to obtain comfort.[76]

Cultivating and Sustaining Compassion and Mindful Practice

Self-care practices

Acute health care settings are stressful environments for the people who work in them. Staff working in critical care units are subjected to sleep disruption, excessive stimuli, physical exhaustion and moral distress that often result in depression, presenteesim, burnout, and compassion fatigue, which places patients at risk for receiving suboptimal care.[77–82] Skills for recognition and educational intervention have been developed and implemented in these units to prevent this.[77,82] In a randomized controlled pilot, both a therapeutic yoga-based mindfulness-based workplace stress reduction program, showed significantly greater improvements on perceived stress, sleep quality, and the heart rhythm coherence ratio of heart rate variability in participants of both groups. There was no difference in the outcomes of groups who received two different delivery venues of the mindfulness-based intervention (online vs in-person).[83]

SUMMARY

An integrative approach creates healing environments that support patients, families, and health care professionals in acute care settings. Several safe and effective modalities can be used to manage symptoms nonpharmacologically, decrease emotional distress, and improve coping skills. Further research is needed to establish the efficacy of these modalities in larger trials and to clarify dosing. Vigorous research is ongoing as knowledge is gained on their putative mechanisms of action. Mindful use of language enhances the innate healing response improves communication and invites patients and families to participate in their care. Staff should be offered access to skills training to cultivate compassion and mindful practice to enhance both patient care and self-care.

REFERENCES

1. Deng GE, Frenkel M, Cohen L, et al. Evidence-based clinical practice guidelines for integrative oncology: complementary therapies and botanicals. J Soc Integr Oncol 2009;7(3):85–120.
2. Krucoff MW, Crater SW, Gallup D, et al. Music, imagery, touch, and prayer as adjuncts to interventional cardiac care: the Monitoring and Actualisation of Noetic Trainings (MANTRA) II randomised study. Lancet 2005;366(9481):211–7.
3. Seskevich JE, Crater SW, Lane JD, et al. Beneficial effects of noetic therapies on mood before percutaneous intervention for unstable coronary syndromes. Nurs Res 2004;53(2):116–21.
4. Vogel JH, Bolling SF, Costello RB, et al. Integrating complementary medicine into cardiovascular medicine. A report of the American College of Cardiology Foundation Task Force on Clinical Expert Consensus Documents (Writing Committee to Develop an Expert Consensus Document on Complementary and Integrative Medicine). J Am Coll Cardiol 2005;46(1):184–221.
5. Lau U, van Niekerk A. Restorying the self: an exploration of young burn survivors' narratives of resilience. Qual Health Res 2011;21:1165–81.
6. Gabor JY, Cooper AB, Crombach SA, et al. Contribution of the intensive care unit environment to sleep disruption in mechanically ventilated patients and healthy subjects. Am J Respir Crit Care Med 2003;167(5):708–15.
7. Gabor JY, Cooper AB, Hanly PJ. Sleep disruption in the intensive care unit. Curr Opin Crit Care 2001;7(1):21–7.

8. Herdegen JJ. Intensive care unit sleep disruption: can the cycle be restored? Crit Care Med 2002;30(3):709–10.

9. Stuck A, Clark MJ, Connelly CD. Preventing intensive care unit delirium: a patient-centered approach to reducing sleep disruption. Dimens Crit Care Nurs 2011; 30(6):315–20.

10. Mantone J. Tracking ties to infection. As rates of hospital-acquired infections have risen, adding billions in costs, experts view a wide range of remedies. Mod Healthc 2006;36(29):30–1.

11. Lemire JA, Harrison JJ, Turner RJ. Antimicorbial activity of metals: mechanisms, molecular targets and applications. Nat Rev Microbiol 2013;11:371–84.

12. Galib, Barve M, Mashru M, et al. Therapeutic potentials of metals in ancient India: a review through Charaka Samhita. J Ayurveda Integr Med 2011;2(2):55–63.

13. Salgado CD, Sepkowitz KA, John JF, et al. Copper surfaces reduce the rate of healthcare-acquired infections in the intensive care unit. Infect Control Hosp Epidemiol 2013;34(5):479–86.

14. Rai M, Kon K, Ingle A, et al. Broad-spectrum bioactivities of silver nanoparticles: the emerging trends and future prospects. Appl Microbiol Biotechnol 2014;98(5): 1951–61.

15. Lederer JW, Jarvis WR, Thomas L, et al. Multicenter cohort study to assess the impact of a silver-alloy and hydrogel-coated urinary catheter on symptomatic catheter-associated urinary tract infections. J Wound Ostomy Continence Nurs 2014;41(5):473–80.

16. Dossey BM, Keegan L, editors. Holistic nursing. 5th edition. Boston: Jones and Bartlett Publishers; 2009.

17. Kiecolt-Glaser JK, Graham JE, Malarkey WB, et al. Olfactory influences on mood and autonomic, endocrine, and immune function. Psychoneuroendocrinology 2008;33(3):328–39.

18. Warnke PH, Sherry E, Russo PA, et al. Antibacterial essential oils in malodorous cancer patients: clinical observations in 30 patients. Phytomedicine 2006;13(7): 463–7.

19. Sanders C, Diego M, Fernandez M, et al. EEG asymmetry responses to lavender and rosemary aromas in adults and infants. Int J Neurosci 2002;112(11): 1305–20.

20. Wilkinson SM, Love SB, Westcombe AM, et al. Effectiveness of aromatherapy massage in the management of anxiety and depression in patients with cancer: a multicenter randomized controlled trial. J Clin Oncol 2007;25(5):532–9.

21. Buckle J. Clinical aromatherapy: essential oils in practice. 2nd edition. Philadelphia: Churchill Livingstone; 2003.

22. Kon KV, Rai MK. Plant essential oils and their constituents in coping with multidrug-resistant bacteria. Expert Rev Anti Infect Ther 2012;10(7):775–90.

23. Langeveld WT, Veldhuizen EJ, Burt SA. Synergy between essential oil components and antibiotics: a review. Crit Rev Microbiol 2014;40(1):76–94.

24. Fadli M, Saad A, Sayadi S, et al. Antibacterial activity of *Thymus maroccanus* and *Thymus broussonetii* essential oils against nosocomial infection - bacteria and their synergistic potential with antibiotics. Phytomedicine 2012;19(5):464–71.

25. Blackwood B, Thompson G, McMullan R, et al. Tea tree oil (5%) body wash versus standard care (Johnson's Baby Softwash) to prevent colonization with methicillin-resistant *Staphylococcus aureus* in critically ill adults: a randomized controlled trial. J Antimicrob Chemother 2013;68(5):1193–9.

26. Warnke PH, Lott AJ, Sherry E, et al. The ongoing battle against multi-resistant strains: in-vitro inhibition of hospital-acquired MRSA, VRE, *Pseudomonas*, ESBL

E. coli and *Klebsiella* species in the presence of plant-derived antiseptic oils. J Craniomaxillofac Surg 2013;41(4):321–6.

27. Altshuler J, Spoelhof B. Pain, agitation, delirium, and neuromuscular blockade: a review of basic pharmacology, assessment, and monitoring. Crit Care Nurs Q 2013;36(4):356–69.

28. Sawh SB, Selvaraj IP, Danga A, et al. Use of methylnaltrexone for the treatment of opioid-induced constipation in critical care patients. Mayo Clin Proc 2012;87(3): 255–9.

29. Colquhoun D, Novella SP. Acupuncture is theatrical placebo. Anesth Analg 2013; 116(6):1360–3.

30. Zhang Y, Lao L, Chen H, et al. Acupuncture use among American adults: what acupuncture practitioners can learn from National Health Interview Survey 2007? Evid Based Complement Alternat Med 2012;2012:710–50.

31. Highfield ES, Kaptchuk TJ, Ott MJ, et al. Availability of acupuncture in the hospitals of a major academic medical center: a pilot study. Complement Ther Med 2003;11(3):177–83.

32. Lindquist R, Sendelbach S, Windenburg DC, et al. Challenges of implementing a feasibility study of acupuncture in acute and critical care settings. AACN Adv Crit Care 2008;19(2):202–10.

33. Crespin DJ, Griffin KH, Johnson JR, et al. Acupuncture provides short-term pain relief for patients in a total joint replacement program. Pain Med 2015. [Epub ahead of print].

34. Ng SS, Leung WW, Mak TW, et al. Electroacupuncture reduces duration of postoperative ileus after laparoscopic surgery for colorectal cancer. Gastroenterology 2013;144(2):307–13.e1.

35. Chang LH, Hsu CH, Jong GP, et al. Auricular acupressure for managing postoperative pain and knee motion in patients with total knee replacement: a randomized sham control study. Evid Based Complement Alternat Med 2012;2012:528452.

36. Chen HM, Chang FY, Hsu CT. Effect of acupressure on nausea, vomiting, anxiety and pain among post-cesarean section women in Taiwan. Kaohsiung J Med Sci 2005;21(8):341–50.

37. Hjelmstedt A, Shenoy ST, Stener-Victorin E, et al. Acupressure to reduce labor pain: a randomized controlled trial. Acta Obstet Gynecol Scand 2010;89(11):1453–9.

38. Monti DA, Peterson C, Kunkel EJ, et al. A randomized, controlled trial of mindfulness-based art therapy (MBAT) for women with cancer. Psychooncology 2006;15(5):363–73.

39. Broadbent E, Ellis CJ, Gamble G, et al. Changes in patient drawings of the heart identify slow recovery after myocardial infarction. Psychosom Med 2006;68(6): 910–3.

40. Sonke J, Pesata V, Arce L, et al. The effects of arts-in-medicine programming on the medical-surgical work environment. Arts Health 2015;7(1):27–41.

41. O'Shea J, Dodd L, Panayiotou S, et al. Self-induced hypnosis for bilateral ankle arthroscopy. Br J Anaesth 2011;106(2):282.

42. Lang EV, Berbaum KS, Pauker SG. Beneficial effects of hypnosis and adverse effects of empathic attention during percutaneous tumor treatment: when being nice does not suffice. J Vasc Interv Radiol 2008;19(6):897–905.

43. Lang E. A Better patient experience through better communication. J Radiol Nurs 2012;31(4):114–9.

44. Lang EV, Berbaum KS, Faintuch S, et al. Adjunctive self-hypnotic relaxation for outpatient medical procedures: a prospective randomized trial with women undergoing large core breast biopsy. Pain 2006;126(1–3):155–64.

45. Schwab D, Davies D, Bodtker T, et al. A study of efficacy and cost-effectiveness of guided imagery as a portable, self-administered, presurgical intervention delivered by a health plan. Adv Mind Body Med 2007;22(1):8–14.

46. Fulambarker A, Farooki B, Kheir F, et al. Effect of yoga in chronic obstructive pulmonary disease. Am J Ther 2010;19:96–100.

47. Howie-Esquivel J, Lee J, Collier G, et al. Yoga in heart failure patients: a pilot study. J Card Fail 2010;16(9):742–9.

48. Oswal P, Nagarathna R, Ebnezar J, et al. The effect of add-on yogic prana energization technique (YPET) on healing of fresh fractures: a randomized control study. J Altern Complement Med 2011;17(3):253–8.

49. Streeter CC, Whitfield TH, Owen L, et al. Effects of yoga versus walking on mood, anxiety, and brain GABA levels: a randomized controlled MRS study. J Altern Complement Med 2010;16(11):1145–52.

50. Smith MC, Stallings MA, Mariner S, et al. Benefits of massage therapy for hospitalized patients: a descriptive and qualitative evaluation. Altern Ther Health Med 1999;5(4):64–71.

51. Currin J, Meister EA. A hospital-based intervention using massage to reduce distress among oncology patients. Cancer Nurs 2008;31(3):214–21.

52. Shor-Posner G, Hernandez-Reif M, Miguez MJ, et al. Impact of a massage therapy clinical trial on immune status in young Dominican children infected with HIV-1. J Altern Complement Med 2006;12(6):511–6.

53. Rapaport MH, Schettler P, Breese C. A preliminary study of the effects of a single session of Swedish massage on hypothalamic-pituitary-adrenal and immune function in normal individuals. J Altern Complement Med 2010;16(10):1079–88.

54. Morhenn V, Beavin LE, Zak PJ. Massage increases oxytocin and reduces adrenocorticotropin hormone in humans. Altern Ther Health Med 2012;18(6):11–8.

55. Bauer BA, Cutshall SM, Wentworth LJ, et al. Effect of massage therapy on pain, anxiety, and tension after cardiac surgery: a randomized study. Complement Ther Clin Pract 2010;16(2):70–5.

56. Fisher P. What is homeopathy? An introduction. Front Biosci (Elite Ed) 2012;4: 1669–82.

57. Ong CK, Bodeker G, Grundy C, et al. WHO global atlas of traditional, complementary and alternative medicine. Kobe, Japan: WHO Centre for Health Development; 2005.

58. Food and Drug Administration. Food, Drug, and Cosmetic Act of 1938, Pub. L. 103-417, 52 Sta. 1041(1938), as amended and codified in 21 U.S.C.§321(g)(1) (1938). Available at: http://www.fda.gov/ICECI/ComplianceManuals/Compliance PolicyGuidanceManual/ucm074360.htm. Accessed February 27, 2015.

59. Mattson MP. Hormesis defined. Ageing Res Rev 2008;7(1):1–7.

60. Chikramane P, Suresh A, Bellare J, et al. Extreme homeopathic dilutions retain starting materials: a nanoparticulate perspective. Homeopathy 2010;99:231–42.

61. Bell I, Koithan M. A model for homeopathic remedy effects: low dose nanoparticles, allostatic cross-adaptation, and time-dependent sensitization in a complex adaptive system. BMC Complement Altern Med 2012;12:191.

62. Marzotto M, Olioso D, Brizzi M, et al. Extreme sensitivity of gene expression in human SH-SY5Y neurocytes to ultra-low doses of *Gelsemium sempervirens*. BMC Complement Altern Med 2014;14:104.

63. Frass M, Linkesch M, Banyai S, et al. Adjunctive homeopathic treatment in patients with severe sepsis: a randomized, double-blind, placebo-controlled trial in an intensive care unit. Homeopathy 2011;100(1–2):95–100.

64. Frass M, Dielacher C, Linkesch M, et al. Influence of potassium dichromate on tracheal secretions in critically ill patients. Chest 2005;127(3):936–41.
65. Barnes J, Resch KL, Ernst E. Homeopathy for postoperative ileus? A meta-analysis. J Clin Gastroenterol 1997;25(4):628–33.
66. Bellavite P, Conforti A, Marzotto M, et al. Testing homeopathy in mouse emotional response models: pooled data analysis of two series of studies. Evid Based Complement Alternat Med 2012;2012:954374.
67. Magnani P, Conforti A, Zanolin E, et al. Dose-effect study of *Gelsemium sempervirens* in high dilutions on anxiety-related responses in mice. Psychopharmacology (Berl) 2010;210(4):533–45.
68. Peredery O, Persinger MA. Herbal treatment following post-seizure induction in rat by lithium pilocarpine: *Scutellaria lateriflora* (Skullcap), *Gelsemium sempervirens* (Gelsemium) and *Datura stramonium* (Jimson Weed) may prevent development of spontaneous seizures. Phytother Res 2004;18(9):700–5.
69. FitzHenry F, Wells N, Slater V, et al. A randomized placebo-controlled pilot study of the impact of healing touch on fatigue in breast cancer patients undergoing radiation therapy. Integr Cancer 2014;13(2):105–13.
70. Jain S, Mills PJ. Biofield therapies: helpful or full of hype? A best evidence synthesis. Int J Behav Med 2010;17(1):1–16.
71. Jain S, Pavlik D, Distefan J, et al. Complementary medicine for fatigue and cortisol variability in breast cancer survivors: a randomized controlled trial. Cancer 2012;118(3):777–87.
72. Crowe BJ. Toward a new theory of music. Lanham (MD): The Scarecrow Press; 2004.
73. Madison A, Silverman M. The effect of music therapy on relaxation, anxiety, pain perception, and nausea in adult solid organ transplant patients. J Music Ther 2010;47(3):220–32.
74. Craigie FC. Positive spirituality in health care: nine practical approaches to pursuing wholeness for clinicians, Patients and Health Care Organizations. Minneapolis, MN: Mill City Publishing; 2010.
75. Kaptchuk TJ, Friedlander E, Kelley JM, et al. Placebos without deception: a randomized controlled trial in irritable bowel syndrome. PLoS One 2010;5(12):e15591.
76. The Joint Commission. Advancing effective communication, cultural competence, and patient- and family-centered care: a roadmap for hospitals. Oakbrook Terrace, IL: The Joint Commission; 2010.
77. Back AL, Deignan PF, Potter PA. Compassion, compassion fatigue, and burnout: key insights for oncology professionals. Am Soc Clin Oncol Educ Book 2014;e454–9.
78. Hinderer KA, VonRueden KT, Friedmann E, et al. Burnout, compassion fatigue, compassion satisfaction, and secondary traumatic stress in trauma nurses. J Trauma Nurs 2014;21(4):160–9.
79. Houck D. Helping nurses cope with grief and compassion fatigue: an educational intervention. Clin J Oncol Nurs 2014;18(4):454–8.
80. Hunsaker S, Chen HC, Maughan D, et al. Factors that influence the development of compassion fatigue, burnout, and compassion satisfaction in emergency department nurses. J Nurs Scholarsh 2015;47:186–94.
81. Mason VM, Leslie G, Clark K, et al. Compassion fatigue, moral distress, and work engagement in surgical intensive care unit trauma nurses: a pilot study. Dimens Crit Care Nurs 2014;33(4):215–25.

82. Sanso N, Galiana L, Oliver A, et al. Palliative care professionals' inner life: exploring the relationships among awareness, self-care and compassion satisfaction and fatigue, burn out, and coping with death. J Pain Symptom Manage 2015. [Epub ahead of print].

83. Wolever RQ, Bobinet KJ, McCabe K, et al. Effective and viable mind-body stress reduction in the workplace: a randomized controlled trial. J Occup Health Psychol 2012;17(2):246–58.

Palliative Care, Ethics, and the Law in the Intensive Care Unit

Caroline M. Quill, MD, MSHP[a],*, Bernard L. Sussman, MD[b],
Timothy E. Quill, MD[b]

KEYWORDS

- Palliative care • Law • Ethics • Intensive care

KEY POINTS

- Legal, ethical, and palliative issues frequently arise in the care of critically ill patients who may be facing death.
- Withholding and withdrawing life-sustaining therapies, surrogate decision making, and medical futility are frequent scenarios that critical care practitioners encounter.
- Effective communication is a key to avoiding conflict in these domains, and nurses play a key role in such communication.

INTRODUCTION

Approximately 20% of Americans die during or soon after admission to an intensive care unit (ICU).[1] Even for patients who survive, admission to an ICU often involves complex ethical decision making and management of pain and suffering, alongside extremely complex medical management. ICUs have existed in the United States since the 1950s, and over the course of the last half-century have been the setting for many ethical and legal debates in medicine. This article outlines 3 important domains that lie at the intersection of critical care, palliative care, ethics, and the law:

1. Withholding and withdrawing potentially life-sustaining therapies
2. Making decisions for critically ill patients who lack decision-making capacity
3. Approaching cases of perceived futility when patients and/or families still want "everything" done medically

Each domain is centered on an actual clinical scenario, which reviews important principles and precedents that underlie our understanding of how nurses and doctors should approach critically ill patients in the ICU who are likely to be near the end of life.

[a] Pulmonary & Critical Care Medicine, Department of Medicine, University of Rochester Medical Center, 601 Elmwood Avenue, Box 692, Rochester, NY 14642, USA; [b] Palliative Care Medicine, Department of Medicine, University of Rochester Medical Center, 601 Elmwood Avenue, Box 687, Rochester, NY, USA
* Corresponding author.
E-mail address: caroline_quill@urmc.rochester.edu

Crit Care Nurs Clin N Am 27 (2015) 383–394
http://dx.doi.org/10.1016/j.cnc.2015.05.007
0899-5885/15/$ – see front matter © 2015 Elsevier Inc. All rights reserved.
ccnursing.theclinics.com

CASE 1. WITHHOLDING AND WITHDRAWING POTENTIALLY LIFE-SUSTAINING THERAPIES
Case Presentation

A 70-year-old man with advanced chronic obstructive pulmonary disease (COPD) who has been in the hospital receiving systemic steroids, antibiotics, inhaled bronchodilators, diuretics, and supplemental oxygen over the past week for an acute exacerbation without improvement. His oxygen saturation runs between 80% and 90%, and his P_{CO_2} is in the 80s. He rates his dyspnea as averaging 7 on a 10-point scale (0 = none and 10 = extremely severe), and he is on low-dose hydromorphone to lessen his sensation of shortness of breath. He has been "full code" (full cardiopulmonary resuscitation including mechanical ventilation), but his providers fear that if he went onto a ventilator he would never get off.

In brainstorming about alternatives to long-term ventilation if he deteriorates in the near future, the treating medical team identified the following possibilities:

- *Time-limited trial of intubation and mechanical ventilation.*[2] This approach is a possibility for patients with a potentially reversible process such as an acute infection who do not want long-term invasive support or tracheostomy. If they do not respond within an agreed-upon time frame, the expectation set in advance would be that the invasive, potentially life-prolonging therapy would be stopped and the patient would die.
- *Trial of "noninvasive ventilation"* (continuous positive airway pressure or bilevel positive airway pressure [BiPAP]). This option is short of intubation and mechanical ventilation for patients who are "do-not-intubate," but may have a potentially reversible component to their illness or want to stay alive a little longer for a particular event (eg, the arrival of a loved one to "say goodbye" before death).
- *Continue current treatments without escalation of disease-directed therapy if the patient deteriorates.* This option gives the patient more time to respond to current interventions, with simultaneous efforts to palliate uncomfortable symptoms. If the patient improves, treatments are continued and adjusted accordingly. If the patient deteriorates, he or she would transition to the next option:
- *Shift goals to "comfort measures only."*[3] This approach might include continuing current noninvasive medical treatments directed at the patient's COPD because treatments that help his breathing will also be "comfort oriented." It could also include stopping laboratory panels including blood gas monitoring, and initiating more aggressive use of opioids and benzodiazepines to manage his shortness of breath, particularly if it worsens in the near future.

If the patient was already receiving mechanical ventilation and cannot be safely extubated, his additional options would include:

- *Long-term mechanical ventilation and tracheostomy.* The patient would likely have to remain in an acute medical facility until death. There are relatively few nursing facilities or home situations that can manage such patients, who are usually medically fragile and in need of constant monitoring and technical support.
- *"Sink or swim" extubation.*[4] Patients already receiving mechanical ventilation who do not want long-term ventilator support but have a small chance of living for a substantial period of time (usually weeks to months) off the ventilator might choose this option. Here the patient is made as medically stable as possible, and the endotracheal tube and ventilator are then removed with plans to not reintroduce them. In general, opioids and sedatives are minimized during

the withdrawal process as long as there is a reasonable chance of survival, but they are increased if that chance no longer exists and the patient begins to actively die.

- *Ventilator withdrawal with the expectation that the patient will not survive (often called terminal extubation).*[4] In these circumstances, usually whatever analgesics and sedatives already being given are increased by approximately 30% before extubation, and then are increased as needed to relieve increased symptoms if they emerge as the process unfolds. Because terminal extubation is a common procedure and because there are wide variations in how it is approached within and between institutions, it is good policy to develop a protocol for the process within one's institution.

Basic principles underlying these decisions include the following:

- *Discuss options among the interdisciplinary team up front.* Bedside nurses often have unique and important perspectives on the benefits and burdens of treatment because of their time at the bedside caring for the patient and their interactions with the patient's family. The varying perspectives among team members should be integrated into any recommendations that might be made to the patient and family about levels of aggressiveness or limitations to treatment.
- *Comprehensive symptom management.* Whether the primary goal is comfort or living as long as possible, it can be difficult to predict in advance how severe symptoms will be. Because there is such wide variation in the use of opioids and sedatives (ranging from negligent undertreatment of symptoms in a dying patient to overly aggressive use out of proportion to the patient's discomfort), these processes should be overseen by a clinician with experience in symptom palliation. If there are discrepant views about the patient's level of distress, the bedside nurses' perspective should be regularly sought. If the patient's main goal is comfort, referral to hospice care for added support, guidance, and bereavement follow-up should be considered.[3]
- *Aggressive treatment.* When the main goal is continued survival, even if it means having to tolerate some uncomfortable symptoms and indefinite invasive ventilation, any and all potentially effective life-prolonging interventions should be initiated and continued.[5] Every effort should be made to simultaneously palliate any uncomfortable symptoms, but the patient's overarching priorities and goals in terms of life prolongation should not be repeatedly questioned unless there is a major change in his or her condition.
- *Treatment with some limitations in aggressiveness.* Some patients and families will continue searching for a middle ground, trying to think through the risks and benefits of each potential disease-directed intervention, consenting to try some and forgoing others, while trying to simultaneously keep the patient's comfort and dignity in mind. Some of these families want to be involved in all decisions big and small, and others will trust the clinical team to understand their philosophy and act on their behalf.

Case 1 (continued): Once the patient was fully informed about the very low likelihood of getting off a ventilator, he agreed to do not resuscitate (DNR)/do not intubate status. He was willing to try BiPAP at night, and to use it as needed during the day. He stabilized to a degree on this regimen, although because of the BiPAP he was too fragile and medically dependent to live away from the pulmonary step-down unit where he survived for an additional 2 months. He then developed an acute respiratory infection that did not respond to antibiotics. At that time he became markedly symptomatic from dyspnea, fever, and delirium. His family reiterated his desire to not go onto a ventilator, and he was shifted to "comfort measures only" treatment philosophy. He died comfortably within 48 hours.

The palliative care principles and issues in this case were fairly straightforward, although the clinical decision making was at times very challenging, partly because of the number of choices that had to be made:

- Every effort was made to palliate the patient's symptoms and give him a wide range of options no matter which overall approach was taken. Even if he had chosen long-term ventilation including tracheostomy, palliative treatments would still have been part of his treatment.
- The patient and family were informed about the full range of options, using medical knowledge and what was known about the patient's views and values to help guide the process as much as possible.[6] In this case, the clinician clearly and directly recommended against intubation and mechanical ventilation while considering BiPAP as an intermediate step; it later evolved to recommending more aggressive symptom management and eventual withdrawal of the BiPAP. Patients and families need the guidance of experienced clinicians who know their values and have their best interests in mind.
- BiPAP can be a temporizing palliative measure, but often in patients with end-stage cardiopulmonary diseases BiPAP can be continually needed to stay alive. In such a context, BiPAP may also prolong the final stages of a very difficult dying process, aggravating without improving the quality of life.[7] It also has the disadvantage of requiring patients and their families to "give up" on yet one more treatment before they die.

The ethical issues in this case were also relatively straightforward, although their implementation was at times complex:

- The patient and his family needed to be directly involved in all major decisions, albeit guided by the recommendations of a clinician who was experienced and aware of the patient's values and priorities.[6]
- Although stopping a ventilator once started is "ethically equivalent" to not starting it, it would be better to say that both are permissible based on the right to bodily integrity. Not going on the ventilator in the first place was a big decision, and saved the patient, family, and staff from the added burden of potentially stopping it with a terminal extubation.
- The use of opioids to treat shortness of breath is often justified by the rule of double effect, which puts weight on "intended" versus "foreseen" consequences of an action.[8,9] Early on, doses of opioids were minimized to lessen the risk of respiratory depression and carbon dioxide retention (very real risks in this case), but later as he was actively dying and his dyspnea was more extreme, higher doses were justified even though it could be foreseen that they could possibly contribute to an earlier death. In this case, the risks taken were "proportionate" to the degree of suffering being treated, and the intention of the increased dose was not to hasten death—additional requirements of the rule.

The legal issues raised by this case are largely settled in the United States:

- Patients have the right to consent to or refuse any medical treatment based on the right to bodily integrity.[10] That right would include both potentially effective disease-directed therapies and palliative treatments.

- The line of decision-making authority used in this case also is largely settled legally in the United States.[11,12] It would include, in the following hierarchical order
  1. Competent patient making decisions for himself or herself
  2. Surrogate decision maker named by the patient (health care proxy), ideally using what is known of the patient's views and values as a guide ("substituted judgment": making surrogate decisions using what is known about the incapacitated patient's views and values rather than those of the surrogate decision maker)
  3. Surrogate decision maker from a hierarchical list that may vary from state to state (spouse, living adult children, parents, sibling, close relative, close friend) ideally using substituted judgment. If the patient's wishes are not known or knowable, surrogate decision makers should be guided (along with the clinicians working with them) by the patient's best interests.
- In this case, the patient made his own decisions until the very end, when his family used substituted judgment to assist the medical team with the final decisions.

CASE 2. MAKING DECISIONS FOR CRITICALLY ILL PATIENTS WHO LACK DECISION-MAKING CAPACITY
Case Presentation

An elderly woman with an unknown medical history presents to the Emergency Department after she was found unconscious on the floor at home by a concerned neighbor. On presentation she is febrile, hypoxemic, and hypotensive. The medical team attempts to ask her questions regarding her wishes with respect to intubation and resuscitation, but her responses are incoherent. No family is available to assist with decision making. A plan is made to intubate but, while preparing for the procedure, the patient suffers a cardiac arrest. She is intubated and successfully resuscitated after 2 rounds of cardiopulmonary resuscitation (CPR). Initial labs drawn before the arrest reveal a pH of 7.1 and a lactate of 8.

In most hospitals in the United States, it is assumed that unless a patient's explicit wishes to the contrary are known, mechanical ventilation and CPR should be provided as the default option to all patients at the time of cardiopulmonary arrest. Although review of an individual hospital's policy regarding mechanical ventilation and CPR is important, the providers in this case are ethically and legally justified in performing intubation and CPR for a critically ill patient who lacks decision-making capacity, and is without a surrogate clearly declining the procedure on the patients' behalf or previously expressed advance directives limiting aggressive care.

CPR and defibrillation therapy were introduced as potentially life-saving interventions in the 1960s. Soon thereafter, American hospitals typically required that CPR be provided to patients suffering cardiac arrest, both inside and outside the ICU. In 1974, the American Medical Association (AMA) proposed that DNR decisions be documented in the medical record and acknowledged that CPR may not be indicated in certain situations.[13] In response to most inpatients requiring CPR not surviving to hospital discharge,[14] the 1980s saw the evolution of the so-called slow code whereby physicians delayed CPR or provided ineffective resuscitation for patients suffering a cardiac arrest whom they did not consider would benefit from such therapy. Slow codes and other similar interventions were in many ways a covert (albeit unethical because of the deception involved) protest to universal resuscitation policies. Although a slow code is clearly a violation of patient trust, this also represented an evolving notion that some patients or their surrogate decision makers should not be offered CPR when it is clearly ineffective.

Case 2 (continued): The patient is admitted to the ICU, where her hemodynamics initially stabilize with the help of antibiotics for presumed septic shock, volume resuscitation, and vasopressors. Her mental status improves modestly, and she is able to follow simple commands while on the ventilator. Over the next several days her kidney function worsens, attributed to septic shock and hypotension. Because of refractory acidosis and volume overload, the medical team wonders about initiating hemodialysis. The patient is unable to express her wishes regarding hemodialysis or other aggressive modes of care, but 2 daughters who live out of town are identified. Neither daughter is aware of any prewritten advance directive or living will, and no one has been officially identified as a health care proxy. The patient's husband died the previous year after a stroke. The medical providers ask the daughters to help decide whether to pursue hemodialysis.

As in the first case, palliative care principles in this case are straightforward. The patient's daughters will have 3 basic options: (1) to continue all aggressive care including mechanical ventilation and hemodialysis; (2) to place some limits on care (such as not initiating hemodialysis); or (3) to transition to fully comfort-focused care, which may include withdrawing mechanical ventilation. Regardless of which option is selected, every effort should be made by providers to palliate symptoms, particularly pain, anxiety, dyspnea, and delirium, all of which are common in critically ill patients. Only rarely will surrogates decline appropriate pain and symptom management for their loved ones. Such cases warrant involvement of palliative care specialists and perhaps ethics consultation to better understand the dynamics and concerns underlying such requests.

Substituted Judgment and the Law

Decisionally capable patients have the right to request or refuse any potentially effective life-prolonging therapy, including hemodialysis, mechanical ventilation, and CPR.[15–17] If patients are not capable of autonomous decision making, their surrogate decision makers are empowered to decide as they believe the patient would, using substituted judgment when possible, and using the patient's best interests if the relevant views and values of the patient cannot be ascertained.[18–20] It is estimated that 60% to 80% of critically ill patients lack decision-making capacity at some point during their ICU stay.[21] As a result, clinicians frequently rely on surrogate decision makers.

Much of our understanding of how medical decisions are to be made for incompetent patients stems from several legal precedents:

- *In re Quinlan*[22]: A 1976 case of Karen Ann Quinlan, a young woman who suffered a cardiac arrest under uncertain circumstances at the age of 21. When she was determined to be in a persistent vegetative state after several months, her father sought guardianship with the intent to remove her from mechanical ventilation. His request for guardianship was denied, and the treating hospital and physicians sought a restraining order against Mr Quinlan, believing that removing the ventilator amount to euthanasia. When the case was ultimately appealed to the supreme court of New Jersey, it was ruled that her father, through substituted judgment, could request that the ventilator be removed. This case established that surrogates could refuse mechanical ventilation on behalf of incapacitated patients using what is known of the patient's views and values. Ms Quinlan's ventilator was removed but she did not die as anticipated. She lived for another 8 years supported by a feeding tube before she eventually died in 1985.
- *In re Cruzan*[23,24]: Nancy Cruzan was a young woman in a persistent vegetative state as a result of an automobile accident. She was receiving tube feedings to

sustain her life but was on no other life-sustaining therapies. Based on their knowledge of her preexisting wishes, her parents requested that her tube feeds be discontinued and that she be "allowed to die." The Supreme Court ruled that patients have a constitutional right to refuse life-sustaining treatments including hydration and nutrition, but states could set standards for how much evidence is required for surrogates to make such decisions (Missouri had a "clear and convincing evidence" requirement for such decisions, which the family ultimately was able to meet based on Ms Cruzan's prior statements and values).

- *The Patient Self-Determination Act*[25]: Passed by Congress in 1990, the act requires that federally funded health care institutions inquire about advance directives on admission to the hospital and that patient preferences should be a part of the medical record.

Ethical Principles Involved in Cases of Substituted Judgment

Most decision-making guidance is grounded in the ethical principle of respect for patient autonomy. A consensus statement from the Society of Critical Care Medicine in 1990 states that the wishes of an informed adult patient with intact decision-making capacity should guide virtually all treatment decisions in the ICU.[26] Beneficence, non-maleficence, and respect for autonomy all guide basic decision making in the ICU. These principles may come into conflict when patient or family wishes conflict with each other or with medical providers' impressions of what is best for a patient. In the United States patient autonomy is often the dominant ethical principle, and this includes respect for substituted judgment (in essence autonomy by proxy), although there is certainly variation among countries and cultures.

A few circumstances warrant special attention.

- *Decision making for an incapacitated patient who has no surrogate decision maker.* This scenario is encountered frequently in ICUs, with one study estimating that 16% of patients admitted to a single-center medical ICU lacked both decision-making capacity and a surrogate decision maker.[27] Professional society guidelines have varied recommendations for such patients, with many, including the AMA and the American College of Physicians, recommending consideration of judicial review. Despite these recommendations, a 2007 multi-center ICU study by White and colleagues[28] found that approximately 5% of deaths in ICUs occurred in incapacitated patients without a surrogate decision maker or an advance directive. Clinicians used a variety of means to make such decisions including hospital review, consensus decision making by the interprofessional ICU team alone, or consensus building with the input of other independent clinicians and ethicists. Only 1 of 37 cases used court review.
- *Decision making for a patient with developmental disabilities.* There is substantial regional, national, and international variation on how to make decisions for patients with developmental disabilities. In New York State, for example, persons with developmental disabilities who have been associated with the Office of People with Developmental Disabilities, even those with family support doing their best to represent the patient's best interests, will have review and oversight by agents of state agencies acting on their behalf if limitations on life-sustaining therapy (LST) are being considered; this is stipulated in New York State's Family Health Care Decisions Act.[29] If a patient with a developmental disability lacks capacity to make decisions, a legal guardian, if formally established through the courts, would be recognized as surrogate decision maker, even when an actively involved spouse, parent, or other family member who is not the legal

guardian is available. Familiarity with local and regional regulations when dealing with this special population is recommended.

CASE 3. APPROACHING CASES OF PERCEIVED FUTILITY WHEN PATIENTS AND FAMILIES WANT "EVERYTHING" DONE
Case Presentation

A 50-year-old man with a history of lung cancer with skeletal metastases suffers a cardiac arrest at home and undergoes extended out-of-hospital CPR. When hospitalized he has a serum sodium of 100. Correction of his hyponatremia does not alter his persistent coma. He is dependent on mechanical ventilation. Neurologic evaluation confirms global hypoxic brain injury. Prognosis for neurologic improvement is thought to be negligible. When the patient develops evidence of inoperable bowel perforation, peritonitis, and sepsis, his family is approached to discuss goals of care, and a recommendation for withdrawal of LST. The patient's living will identifies his sister as health care proxy and stipulates that he wants no limitations on LST including CPR and mechanical ventilation. The patient's sister and family understand his grim prognosis but feel strongly that his wishes should be respected. Unexpectedly he survives his bowel perforation and sepsis without surgery. After weeks of a stalemate, critical care clinicians become increasingly frustrated and at times angry that they cannot discontinue what seems to them to be futile medical treatment.

Ethical Conflict Over Medical Futility in the Intensive Care Unit

Medical futility emerged in the 1980s as a prominent bioethical controversy. Nowhere was this conflict more evident than in medical and surgical ICUs, where once unimagined treatments were extending lives of patients without hope of independence from intensive medical care or survival to leave the hospital. Ethical authorization for physicians to unilaterally discontinue treatments perceived to be futile was championed by some and rejected by others.[30–32] Despite failure to establish consensus regarding a definition of futility, the controversy continues to smolder today.[33–35] Medical futility has been criticized as a subterfuge that asserts physicians' values over those of patients and families. Still, there is recognition that nurses and doctors may feel morally compromised by requirements to continue invasive treatments that cannot achieve goals that they consider in a patient's best interest.[32,34,36–38]

Understanding the Ethical Conflict

Futile is defined in the *Oxford English Dictionary* as "incapable of producing any result"; a secondary definition is "lacking in purpose." Much of the confusion and disagreement about medical futility is perhaps rooted in the different meanings of these definitions. The first definition addresses what ought to be objective and measurable. Schneiderman and colleagues[31] proposed identification of 100 consecutive cases of medical treatment that proved useless as grounds for a quantitative determination of futility. This standard has been found unworkable, in part because of the variability of clinical circumstances in specific cases. More centrally, the concept of usefulness is a value-laden term that needs to be understood in the context of goals of treatment. An understanding of patient and family values is all the more important in appeals to qualitative criteria seeking to justify claims of medical futility.[30,32,34]

The second definition of futile ("lacking in purpose") directly concerns values. Perceptions of purpose are inherently matters imbued with personal preference and conviction. Determination that our patient was not a surgical candidate was based on a medical judgment that surgery was unsafe in his medical condition. Evaluating the benefits of surgery for him is appropriately an issue of medical expertise and is fundamental to a clinician's professional integrity. Deciding whether continued LST for him has purpose is a judgment that invokes the values and convictions of the patient and his family. When there is disagreement over the value of treatment, respect for patients and families requires that their autonomous choices be honored.

The ethical issues in this case are reflected in the opposing viewpoints of the critical care team and the patient's family.

- *The provider's view.* Clashes in the ICU over perceived futile medical care commonly mask an underlying conflict about goals of care and the purpose of achievable outcomes. The ICU team saw that the patient would never regain consciousness. Continuing LST would require tracheostomy and other procedures that would expose him to risk without benefit, a potential violation of the principle of nonmaleficence. Underlying their perception of futility was awareness of the patient's metastatic lung cancer and the potential for future suffering. Our patient would never recover consciousness or be able to leave the hospital; hence, any LST was futile in our view.
- *The family's perspective.* The patient's family saw both purpose and value in his continued life support. His living will had been completed with awareness of his metastatic cancer. The sister did not question his prognosis as explained to her. She felt, however, that continuing LST fulfilled her obligation to honor her brother's wishes. To limit her brother's medical treatment would constitute a subversion of his wishes, choices that he had confirmed in conversation with her and in writing. Although she could do nothing to alter her brother's prognosis, she felt that she had the ability and responsibility to safeguard his choices. When asked to consider whether her brother had anticipated his current circumstance when he gave advance direction regarding LST, his sister struggled but ultimately, with the consensus of family, decided that treatment should continue. Repeated efforts to change her decision resulted in a strained relationship with the ICU team, and family members perceived that they were being pressured to abandon their duty.

Palliative care issues in this case are reflected in the ICU nursing experience. Attention to patient suffering and strategies to resolve disagreement over futility reflect both ethical and palliative care priorities:

- *Futility and moral distress.* Perceived futility is central to the moral distress and professional frustration documented to be extensive within the ranks of critical care nurses.[36,37] Hamric and Blackhall[36] have demonstrated that nurses more often experience moral distress in the ICU than do physicians. The most common scenarios associated with moral distress involve feeling pressure to provide life-sustaining treatments for patients who are dying or to engage in medical treatments that serve only to prolong the dying process. Treatment in these circumstances, as in our patient, is perceived as futile.
- The specific moral struggle of ICU nurses in cases of perceived futility has been explained as a consequence of the "hands-on" role of nurses in the ICU. Their abiding presence at the patient's bedside makes them witnesses to what they consider patient suffering. Furthermore, they are responsible for fulfilling orders that they have not initiated and see as harmful, imposing treatments on their patients they would never choose for themselves or their own family members. Too often critical care nurses lack direct participation in discussions of end-of-

life issues with patients and their families. Nurses are frequently not present at the bedside for family meetings when physicians discuss goals of care, and may only learn the bottom-line results of these discussions rather than the story behind decisions to continue LST. Excluded from active participation in the process of listening and discussion, nurses are likewise excluded from the exchanges that might transform their perception of ethically incomprehensible choices into insight, if not agreement.

- *Avoiding and resolving conflict over futility*. Although enthusiasm for unilateral physician action based on claims of medical futility has waned,[30] a consensus regarding approaches to avoid and resolve conflicts over perceived benefits of care in the ICU has emerged. Examination of most futility arguments reveals disagreement over goals of care and values. Efforts to identify and resolve these disagreements begin with questions that ask about the patient and his values. Attentive listening to the patient or the family is fundamental to hopes for resolving and preventing stand-offs. Clear communication over time may contribute to a relationship of trust rather than suspicion. The family may come to recognize that their loved one is in fact dying and that continuing LST will not achieve their goals.[34,37] As already discussed, agreement on time limited trials of LST may help resolve an impasse. ICU teams have an obligation to discuss and explain why they think continued LST is not in a patient's best interest. Offering medical recommendations should not, however, be the only communication from the critical care team. If the family does not feel pressured by doctors and nurses who want them to stop LST, they may come to reconsider their decisions. Irrespective of what decision is made regarding aggressive, disease-directed therapy, every effort to palliate the patient's symptoms should be made.

Appeals to legal action are rare but may be considered if disputes remain entrenched.

- There will be circumstances when these conflicts remain unresolved. Understanding that bioethics and medical professionalism emphasize respect for the autonomy of patients and families may make these stand-offs more tolerable. There can be professional fulfillment in honoring the integrity and self-determination of our patients and families just as we would want our own choices to be honored, even if mistaken. Processes for resolving entrenched conflicts over clearly unavailing treatments have been developed.[38] The Texas Advance Directives Act is one such effort.[39] Appeal to the due process and impartiality of a court decision is a last resort that is rarely used. When it is, nearly all judicial decisions have favored the authority of patients and their surrogates to choose their own goals of medical care.[30]

SUMMARY

Withholding and withdrawing LST, surrogate decision making, and perceived medical futility are 3 classic examples in which palliative care, ethics, and the law intersect in the ICU. An understanding of the principles that dictate the basic management in these cases is imperative for all critical care practitioners. Frequent and effective communication between families and providers, and among providers of all bedside disciplines, is pivotal to avoiding conflicts in these complex cases. Despite their pivotal role at the center of critical care and their often close relationship with patients and families, nurses are often excluded from direct participation in end-of-life decision making. Knowledge of the ethical, legal, and palliative principles that are involved in such decision making will make nursing participation in such decision making ever more valuable.

REFERENCES

1. Angus DC, Barnato AE, Linde-Zwirble WT, et al. Use of intensive care at the end of life in the United States: an epidemiologic study. Crit Care Med 2004;32(3): 638–43.
2. Quill TE, Holloway R. Time-limited trials near the end of life. JAMA 2011;306(13): 1483–4.
3. Lynn J. Perspectives on care at the close of life. Serving patients who may die soon and their families: the role of hospice and other services. JAMA 2001; 285(7):925–32.
4. Kirschner KL, Kerkhoff TR, Butt L, et al. 'I don't want to live this way, doc. Please take me off the ventilator and let me die'. PM R 2011;3(10):968–75.
5. Quill TE, Arnold R, Back AL. Discussing treatment preferences with patients who want "everything". Ann Intern Med 2009;151(5):345–9.
6. Quill TE, Brody H. Physician recommendations and patient autonomy: finding a balance between physician power and patient choice. Ann Intern Med 1996; 125(9):763–9.
7. Quill CM, Quill TE. Palliative use of noninvasive ventilation: navigating murky waters. J Palliat Med 2014;17(6):657–61.
8. Quill TE. Principle of double effect and end-of-life pain management: additional myths and a limited role. J Palliat Med 1998;1(4):333–6.
9. Quill TE, Dresser R, Brock DW. The rule of double effect—a critique of its role in end-of-life decision making. N Engl J Med 1997;337(24):1768–71.
10. Sullivan MD, Youngner SJ. Depression, competence, and the right to refuse life-saving medical treatment. Am J Psychiatry 1994;151(7):971–8.
11. Brock DW. What is the moral authority of family members to act as surrogates for incompetent patients? Milbank Q 1996;74(4):599–618.
12. Lang F, Quill T. Making decisions with families at the end of life. Am Fam Physician 2004;70(4):719–23.
13. Standards for cardiopulmonary resuscitation (CPR) and emergency cardiac care (ECC). V. Medicolegal considerations and recommendations. JAMA 1974; 227(7 Suppl):864–8.
14. Bedell SE, Delbanco TL, Cook EF, et al. Survival after cardiopulmonary resuscitation in the hospital. N Engl J Med 1983;309(10):569–76.
15. Prendergast TJ, Luce JM. Increasing incidence of withholding and withdrawal of life support from the critically ill. Am J Respir Crit Care Med 1997;155(1):15–20.
16. Brody H, Campbell ML, Faber-Langendoen K, et al. Withdrawing intensive life-sustaining treatment—recommendations for compassionate clinical management. N Engl J Med 1997;336(9):652–7.
17. Teno JM, Fisher E, Hamel MB, et al. Decision-making and outcomes of prolonged ICU stays in seriously ill patients. J Am Geriatr Soc 2000;48(5 Suppl):S70–4.
18. Karlawish JH, Quill T, Meier DE. A consensus-based approach to providing palliative care to patients who lack decision-making capacity. ACP-ASIM End-of-Life Care Consensus Panel. American College of Physicians-American Society of Internal Medicine. Ann Intern Med 1999;130(10):835–40.
19. Miller DK, Coe RM, Hyers TM. Achieving consensus on withdrawing or withholding care for critically ill patients. J Gen Intern Med 1992;7(5):475–80.

20. Kassirer JP. Adding insult to injury. Usurping patients' prerogatives. N Engl J Med 1983;308(15):898–901.
21. Girard TD, Pandharipande PP, Ely EW. Delirium in the intensive care unit. Crit Care 2008;12(Suppl 3):S3.
22. In re Quinlan, 755 A2A 647 (NJ), cert denied, 429 70 NJ 10, 355 A2d 647 (1976).
23. Cruzan v. Harmon, 760 SW 2d 408 (Mo, 1988) (en banc).
24. Cruzan v. Director, Missouri Dept. of Health. 110 S ct 2841 (1990).
25. Omnibus Budget Reconciliation Act of 1990. Public Law No. 101–508.
26. Consensus report on the ethics of foregoing life-sustaining treatments in the critically ill. Task Force on Ethics of the Society of Critical Care Medicine. Crit Care Med 1990;18(12):1435–9.
27. White DB, Curtis JR, Lo B, et al. Decisions to limit life-sustaining treatment for critically ill patients who lack both decision-making capacity and surrogate decision-makers. Crit Care Med 2006;34(8):2053–9.
28. White DB, Curtis JR, Wolf LE, et al. Life support for patients without a surrogate decision maker: who decides? Ann Intern Med 2007;147(1):34–40.
29. Available at: http://www.nysarc.org/files/2213/8478/2747/17R_-_OPWDD_Putting_People_First_Brochure_HEALTH_CARE_CHOICES_-_Feb_2012.pdf. Accessed June 15, 2015.
30. Helft PR, Siegler M, Lantos J. The rise and fall of the futility movement. N Engl J Med 2000;343(4):293–6.
31. Schneiderman LJ, Jecker NS, Jonsen AR. Medical futility: its meaning and ethical implications. Ann Intern Med 1990;112(12):949–54.
32. Truog RD, Brett AS, Frader J. The problem with futility. N Engl J Med 1992; 326(23):1560–4.
33. Youngner SJ. Who defines futility? JAMA 1988;260(14):2094–5.
34. Determeyer L, Brody H. Medical futility: content in the context of care. In: Quill TE, Miller FG, editors. Palliative care and ethics. Oxford (United Kingdom): Oxford University Press; 2014. p. 199–208.
35. Burns JP, Truog RD. Futility: a concept in evolution. Chest 2007;132(6):1987–93.
36. Hamric AB, Blackhall LJ. Nurse-physician perspectives on the care of dying patients in intensive care units: collaboration, moral distress, and ethical climate. Crit Care Med 2007;35(2):422–9.
37. Workman S, McKeever P, Harvey W, et al. Intensive care nurses' and physicians' experiences with demands for treatment: some implications for clinical practice. J Crit Care 2003;18(1):17–21.
38. Medical futility in end-of-life care: report of the council on ethical and judicial affairs. JAMA 1999;281(10):937–41.
39. White DB, Pope TM. The courts, futility, and the ends of medicine. JAMA 2012; 307(2):151–2.

Priorities for Evaluating Palliative Care Outcomes in Intensive Care Units

Marie Bakitas, DNSc, CRNP, ACHPN, FAAN[a],*,
J. Nicholas Dionne-Odom, PhD, RN[a], Arif Kamal, MD, MHS[b],
Jennifer M. Maguire, MD[c]

KEYWORDS

- Outcome measures • Evaluation • Intensive care unit • Palliative care
- Performance measures

KEY POINTS

- Palliative care delivery in the intensive care unit (ICU) is growing and is increasingly accepted as an essential component of comprehensive care for the wide array of critically ill patients cared for in ICUs.
- Typical ICU outcome measures have often focused on reducing mortality and length of stay; these are less often considered traditional targets of palliative care.
- Multiple perspectives and domains must be taken into account when measuring ICU outcomes.
- Most ICU palliative care outcomes research has focused on communication.
- Future measurement of ICU outcomes should expand beyond length of stay and costs and focus to a greater extent on patient-centered and family-centered outcomes.

INTRODUCTION

Since the landmark SUPPORT (Study to Understand Prognosis and Preferences for Outcomes and Risks of Treatments) study,[1] significant intensive care unit (ICU) quality-of-care issues (eg, inadequate physician communication, care not matched to patients' goals and preferences, pain, patient and family distress) have been

[a] School of Nursing, Division of Geriatrics, Gerontology, and Palliative Care, University of Alabama at Birmingham, NB 2M019C, 1701 University Boulevard, Birmingham, AL 35233, USA; [b] Division of Medical Oncology, Duke Palliative Care, Duke Clinical Research Institute, Duke University, 2400 Pratt Street, #8043, Durham, NC 27710, USA; [c] Division of Pulmonary Diseases and Critical Care Medicine, University of North Carolina – Chapel Hill, Bioinformatics Building, Suite 4124, Campus Box 7020, Chapel Hill, NC 27599, USA
* Corresponding author. NB 2M019C, 1720 2nd Avenue, South, Birmingham, AL 35294-1210.
E-mail address: mbakitas@uab.edu

Crit Care Nurs Clin N Am 27 (2015) 395–411
http://dx.doi.org/10.1016/j.cnc.2015.05.001
0899-5885/15/$ – see front matter © 2015 Elsevier Inc. All rights reserved.

documented. In 1997[2] and 2014,[3] the Institute of Medicine issued reports further highlighting these concerns, suggesting that although some progress has been made, issues surrounding advance care planning, communication, and lack of incentives to provide high quality end of life care persist, especially for patients who die in ICUs. In addition, an under-recognized consequence of poor quality of care in patients dying in ICUs is the moral distress experienced by the nurses, physicians, and other members of the care team who care for these patients.[4,5]

One widely suggested solution to the many care quality challenges in seriously ill ICU patients has been the integration of palliative care.[6] Via a variety of different models, palliative care is growing and is increasingly accepted as an essential component of comprehensive care for critically ill patients, regardless of diagnosis or prognosis.[7] Models of integrating palliative care services, such as initiating consults by palliative care specialists via triggers[8] or improving the palliative care skills of ICU clinicians,[9] or a combination, have been recommended.[10] Triggers for palliative care in a surgical ICU (SICU) identified by a clinician Delphi study included: family request; futility declared by the medical team; family disagreement with the medical team, the patient's advance directive, or each other lasting greater than 7 days; death expected during the same SICU stay; and SICU stay greater than 1 month.[11] With such triggers, some suggest that up to 1 in 7 ICU patients should be seen by palliative care.[12]

Several benefits from palliative care integration have already been noted. For example, early evidence shows reductions in hospital and ICU lengths of stay without an increase in mortality.[13] Reduced ICU use and length of stay has also resulted in reduced charges per patient, typically because of fewer invasive interventions[14,15] and reduced ICU admission from the general hospital floor.[16] Beneficial family outcomes, including reduced anxiety, depression, and posttraumatic stress disorder, have also been noted.[17,18]

However, unlike organized efforts to evaluate ICU care quality generally, evaluation of the impact of palliative care on outcomes is still in the early stages, although recent advances, such as organized quality improvement initiatives[19,20] and a potential framework on which to comprehensively evaluate ICU palliative care outcomes (**Fig. 1**),[21] are notable. This article discusses the context of ICU palliative outcomes, current methods of assessing palliative care quality outcomes, prospective trials that have attempted to measure selected palliative care outcomes in ICUs, and future directions.

THE CONTEXT OF MEASURING INTENSIVE CARE UNIT PALLIATIVE CARE OUTCOMES

Examination of palliative care outcomes in the ICU begins with understanding the context of the measurement environment; that is, the patients and settings to be studied. More patients are receiving care in a variety of medical, surgical, and subspecialty ICUs than ever before as therapies for chronic and acute illness are increasing.[22] The increasing number of ICU admissions has driven the call for increasing integration of palliative care, especially for patients with end-of-life and symptom management concerns. In particular, Teno and colleagues[23] found that although more Medicare beneficiaries aged 65 yeas and older are dying at home rather than in a hospital, ICU stays in the last month of life are increasing; decedents experiencing an ICU stay in the last months of life increased from 24.3% in 2000 to 29.2% in 2009. Reports from the Dartmouth Atlas of Health Care reinforce these trends. In chronically ill Medicare patients[24,25] from 2003 to 2007 there was an increase in the number of ICU days in the last 6 months of life. In addition, although there was a decrease nationally in the percentage of patients with cancer[24] dying in hospital between 2003 and 2007, there was an increase in those with an ICU stay during the last month of life.[26]

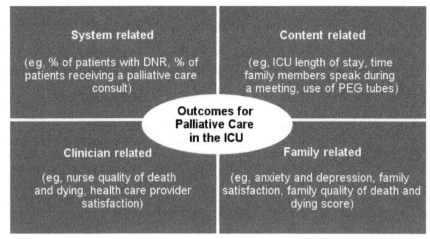

Fig. 1. Potential domains of palliative care ICU outcomes. DNR, do not resuscitate. PEG, percutaneous endoscopic gastrostomy. (*From* Aslakson RA, Bridges JF. Assessing the impact of palliative care in the intensive care unit through the lens of patient-centered outcomes research. Curr Opin Crit Care 2013;19(5):507; with permission.)

Structure among ICU settings varies widely across hospitals. Unit size, volume of admissions, and staffing ratios account in part for this variation. A small hospital with few ICU beds and no intermediate care unit without a dedicated intensivist may have a low-acuity ICU comprising an overflow of patients needing telemetry or postoperative patients to be extubated. More severely ill patients may be transferred to a hospital with greater expertise. A hospital with a cardiac transplant program is likely to have significantly different technologies and staffing ratios. Increasingly, telemedicine[27] with e-ICUs (electronic ICUs) staffed with off-site intensivists are being developed, adding another type of ICU to the mix. Similarly, the availability of palliative care expertise also varies greatly, from a formal palliative care consult team in a tertiary ICU to primary physicians with some palliative care training admitting their patients to the local ICU. This variation dictates a wide range of practices, thus defining palliative care practices and principles is essential for determining the measurement standard for high-quality critical care.

Furthermore, patients in ICUs are one of the most heterogeneous populations in the hospital. ICU admissions range from patients with severe illness to those who are chronically critically ill. Some patients are on extreme lifesaving/life-prolonging technologies such as extracorporeal membrane oxygenation, whereas others are in the ICU for less than 24 hours on an insulin infusion to correct increased blood glucose levels. Patients frequently have prolonged ICU stays and can even require multiple transfers among different levels of critical care (eg, between long-term acute care hospitals or subspecialty ICUs). This diverse population poses unique challenges to implementing and measuring the outcomes of any new or developing expansions on any service line including palliative care.

WHICH OUTCOMES TO MEASURE?

Measuring and reporting outcomes related to the quality and effectiveness of palliative care delivery has become an important component of measuring ICU care. In measuring complex care, key considerations must be given to choosing the priority outcomes of interest, the methodology with which data are collected and analyzed, and the reporters of that information. Similar to the contrasts between research and quality improvement, in which the former requires systematic investigation that leads to conclusions that can be generalized outside of the organization in which the study occurred.[28] Important differences must be noted when outcome measurements are designed to address more local aspects of quality of care. Some important considerations when selecting outcomes measures for research and quality improvement are reviewed here.

Critical care and palliative care have historically focused on differing outcomes, with occasional areas of overlap. For example, critical care evaluation priorities have historically focused on biological outcomes (eg, pH, central venous oxygen concentration), illness severity (eg, APACHE [Acute Physiology and Chronic Health Evaluation] scores), and patient-level use outcomes (eg, in-hospital mortality, ventilator-free days) (Table 1).[29,30] In contrast, palliative care clinical trials have typically examined patient experiences with care (eg, health-related quality of life, patient satisfaction), physical aspects of care (eg, pain, nausea), and emotional well-being (eg, depression, anxiety). The National Consensus Project Clinical Practice Guidelines domains represent a framework within which to consider important outcomes of palliative care[31] (Table 2). Recently, there has been a movement by palliative investigators to measure outcomes related to medical resource use, like 30-day readmission rate,[32] length of stay, and total health care costs.[33,34] Further, a shared focus between palliative and critical care outcomes measurement has included overall survival[35–37]; however, there is no consensus about how to prioritize this outcome and palliative care researchers may not embrace this as a primary outcome for most clinical trials moving forward.

Areas of shared and differing outcomes measurement between the 2 disciplines require careful consideration of historical significance in each field, the target audience when reporting the results of the study, and the policy aim for the study when designing research projects or quality improvement initiatives. As an example, investigators who intend to target the results of a clinical trial testing a communication skills training course to critical care specialists would be wise to choose a mix of ICU-level outcomes (eg, length of stay) alongside the typical outcomes used in palliative care and communications research (eg, family satisfaction, symptom management).[9,38–41]

In addition, the methodology by which the outcomes are collected and analyzed must be considered. For example, with health care quality measures, outcomes measures must reflect an accurate numerator (those who meet the measure; eg, percentage of patients with a health care power of attorney identified) divided by a specific denominator (those eligible for the measure; eg, all patients in the ICU >72 hours).

Table 1
Common outcomes domains measured in critical care

Domain	Examples
Biological	Inflammatory markers, lactate, procalcitonin
Survival	Overall survival, in-hospital mortality
Illness severity	Ventilator-free days, days free of organ dysfunction, new infection, new lung injury
Resource use	Hospital readmission, hospital and ICU length of stay
Patient-reported outcomes	Quality of life, quality of communication
Family-reported outcomes	Satisfaction with care, quality of communication

Table 2
National Consensus Project Clinical Practice Guidelines for Quality Palliative Care domains and examples of measures

Domains	Examples of Measures
Structure and processes of care	Incidence of goals-of-care discussions Presence of interdisciplinary team PCOS Smith-Falvo Patient-Doctor Interaction Scale QUEST FS-ICU Caregiver Strain Index Caregiver Reaction Assessment
Physical aspects of care	McGill Pain Questionnaire Edmonton Symptom Assessment Scale Functional Index of Independence in Activities of Daily Living
Psychological and psychiatric aspects of care	Distress Thermometer TIME After-Death Bereaved Family Interview ICG
Social aspects of care	Quality of Life at the End of Life McGill Quality of Life Questionnaire Meaning in Life Scale
Spiritual, religious, and existential aspects of care	Spiritual Well-Being Scale Spiritual Perspective Scale
Cultural aspects of care	Documented perspectives on death or desires for complementary and alternative medicines
Care of the patient at the end of life	Medical care in the last 48 h of life Actual and preferred site of death QUAL-E QODD
Ethical and legal aspects of life	Access to ethics committees Documentation of the surrogate decision maker PCOS QUAL-E

Abbreviations: FS-ICU, Family Satisfaction in the ICU; ICG, Inventory of Complicated Grief; PCOS, Palliative Care Outcome Scale; QODD, Quality of Death and Dying; QUAL-E, Quality of Life at the End of Life; QUEST, Quality of End-of-Life Care and Satisfaction with Treatment; TIME, Toolkit to Measure End-of-life Care.

This methodology provides the level of an outcome (eg, 85% of patients admitted to the ICU for 72 hours had a health care power of attorney documented in the medical record). Such careful attention allows outcomes to be compared with other organizations (eg, to benchmark), to be reported as part of a study (eg, as the outcome to an intervention), or to be submitted for audit (eg, quality measures as part of bundled payments). Depending on the outcome being measured, the completeness, accuracy, and precision of these data may vary, which ultimately affects the conclusions that can be drawn from the results.

As an example, an ICU study may evaluate changes in Pao_2 through a new ventilation strategy. The reported outcome may be percentage of patients ventilated for at least 72 hours using a lower tidal volume ventilation protocol (denominator) who maintain a Pao_2 of more than 80 mm Hg (numerator). In this case, the outcome, including both the numerator and denominator components, are easily measurable (through regular blood gas monitoring), generally not troubled by missing data (because regular measurements are needed to make clinical decisions and measurement is simple), and is precise (frequent calibration of the instruments).

In contrast, potential measurement challenges in palliative care delivery result from the primarily subjective outcomes that are the targets of palliative care. A trial by Curtis and colleagues[41] evaluated the effect of a communication skills intervention designed for medicine trainees on patient-reported quality of communication (QOC), patient-reported quality of end-of-life care (QEOLC), patient depressive symptoms, and family-reported QOC and QEOLC. Because these were subjective outcomes, involving both the patient and family providing responses, and were collected after the medical care was provided, the study required the investigators to meticulously address potential challenges with missing data, accuracy of measurements, and the precision of the instruments used in the study.

In addition, an important area for consideration when selecting outcomes measures for palliative care integration in the ICU is the understanding of whether the area of investigation is a result of primary or secondary palliative care delivery. There are 2 dominant models by which palliative care is delivered: that which is delivered by critical care clinicians (primary, or sometimes called generalist), or that which involves a specialist as part of a consultative team (secondary or specialist).[42] The latter has been the most common because ICU clinician skills, attitudes, and practices often impede timely palliative care delivery.[43] These barriers begin from medical training,[44] and the downstream practices of ICU attending physicians show wide variation across the United States.[45] However, because of inherent workforce and service provision challenges,[46] not all patients with critical illness can (or should) be evaluated by a secondary, consultative palliative care specialist.

Depending on the delivery model being studied, outcomes measures should be targeted to those most relevant to critical care clinicians' delivery of palliative care, or the introduction of a palliative care specialist. For example, percentage of patients with a family meeting conducted (by anyone) within 7 days of ICU admission may be selected as a basic outcome measure to which all clinicians are subject, versus an 8-domain palliative care assessment performed, including 11-item symptom review for those who perform palliative care consultations as their clinical focus. In the case of evaluation of nursing care outcomes, the evaluation could identify whether a palliative care nurse practitioner specialist ordered an appropriate dose of opioid to manage pain or dyspnea (specialist palliative care process of care outcome), identify the number and frequency of opioid doses administered (generalist bedside nurse process of care outcome), or examine pain or dyspnea relief experienced by the patient in response to opioid medication (specialist/generalist combined outcome).

HOW TO MEASURE INTENSIVE CARE UNIT PALLIATIVE CARE OUTCOMES

The dominant conceptual framework for understanding the relationship between health care quality measures and evaluation of health care quality comes from Avedis Donabedian.[47] He outlined that all quality measures fit into one of 3 categories: structure, process, and outcomes. In this framework, structural measures assess the services, personnel, and resources involved care delivery. For example, clinicians may evaluate the quality of the supportive care services in an ICU by evaluating whether the ICU has a full-time social worker. Process measures evaluate how care is delivered. These measures assess the way in which things are done by the structural components (ie, how does the social worker in the ICU perform an assessment of postdischarge needs?). Of the several thousand quality measures that exist, most are process measures.[48] Outcome measures evaluate the downstream effects of the care processes implemented by the structural aspects of care. This can be thought of as the health state that results from the health care the patient receives. These measures are often reported by patients (eg, satisfaction, symptom relief) or evaluated through electronic health records (eg, survival, pain scores), and are generally presented as frequencies or other descriptive statistics (eg, mean, range).

Measures selected for study typically are process measures. Reasons for this are 3-fold. First, processes are discrete, measurable events. Reviewers can perform chart abstractions, evaluate whether a certain process took place, and compare the frequency of that activity with the total population of patients eligible for that process. Second, process measures do not yield definitive conclusions about the effectiveness of care. They reflect on whether an activity took place, but importantly do not determine the causality between an event and the change in a patient's health state (an outcome). Third, process measures reflect a sense of best practice. Clinicians generally do not avoid process outcomes that are easily discerned from consensus or evidence-driven lists of guidelines, best practices, care pathways, and algorithms. In doing this, clinicians are comfortable in identifying how care should be delivered. However, identifying and measuring the outcomes of clinical importance to the various stakeholders involved in care delivery (ie, patients, caregivers, clinicians, administrators, health systems, and payers) is more challenging and complex.

In 2010 the Center to Advance Palliative Care (CAPC) launched a measurement initiative to centralize measures and provide expert consultation to programs wishing to measure palliative care ICU outcomes (**Box 1** and http://www.capc.org/ipal). The Improving Palliative Care in the ICU (IPAL-ICU) project has undertaken several initiatives to examine ICU palliative care practices. An example of these projects was an extensive examination of care processes: the Agency for Healthcare Research and Quality's National Quality Measures Clearinghouse Care and Communication Bundle.[20] The bundle consists of 9 evidence-based processes of ICU palliative care that are measured through medical record documentation (**Box 2**). In one prospective, observational, multisite study of ICU palliative care, with the exception of pain assessment and management, there was inconsistent or infrequent use of these processes.[20] This finding suggests that integration of palliative care processes into ICUs must be undertaken as an explicit change effort and is unlikely to happen otherwise.

INTENSIVE CARE UNIT PALLIATIVE CARE OUTCOMES RESEARCH AND QUALITY IMPROVEMENT

Aslakson and Bridges[21] proposed another method to conceptualize ICU palliative care outcomes based on the areas addressed by studies to date: systems-related

---

Box 1
The IPAL-ICU (Improving Palliative Care in the ICU) project

The IPAL-ICU project is an initiative of the CAPC that began in 2010. The objective of the IPAL project is to enhance integration and improvement of palliative care in day-to-day ICU practices by creating a central hub for expert consultation and advice, evidence, tools, and resources. As outlined on the CAPC Web site (accessible at http://www.capc.org/ipal), the project has convened a group of nationally recognized experts and leaders who have been developing a catalog of tools and resources that have either been published in the literature or used in established programs. CAPC member organizations can access guidance and tools through the Web site. Additional resources and tools can be shared with CAPC by emailing ipalicu@mssm.edu. Several articles published by the IPAL-ICU project are also available in PubMed or can be obtained at http://www.capc.org/ipal.

Box 2
Care and communication bundle care process performance measures

Identification of medical decision maker

Determination of advanced directive status

Investigation of cardiopulmonary resuscitation preference

Distribution of family information leaflet

Interdisciplinary family meeting conducted

Offer of social work support

Offer of spiritual support

Regular pain assessment

Appropriate pain management

---

areas, content-related areas, clinician-related areas, and family-related areas (**Fig. 1**). Systems-related outcomes are those related to the whole of care (eg, care and communication bundle). Mortality could also be considered an outcome of the entire care delivery system. Content-related outcomes describe the care that is being provided, such as family meetings in which goals of care are discussed. Clinician-related outcomes involve the impact of a project on the nursing or medical staff. For example, educational interventions to improve palliative care skills would evaluate knowledge and skills as a clinician outcome. Family-related outcomes, such as satisfaction with communication, are most often a target of ICU palliative care because most patients in ICUs at end of life are rarely conscious, so the target of care is the family.

Table 3 shows a representative set of 7 prospective studies that have evaluated the impact of palliative care in the ICU.[40,49–53] Although all 7 studies assessed multiple outcomes, the table groups each study into just 1 of the 4 domains described earlier by Aslakson and Bridges.[21] Four studies[40,51–53] focused on systems-related outcomes, such as the percentage of patients with do-not-resuscitate orders, goals-of-care and prognostic discussions within 24 hours of admission, and family meetings within 72 hours. All 4 used a multicomponent approach. For example, Penrod and colleagues[53] reported on an intervention that consisted of ICU nurse team training, auditing and performance feedback, distribution of improvement tools, and monthly team meetings. Across all 4 of these studies, most of the desired outcomes were accomplished. One study, by Norton and colleagues,[54] focused on Aslakson and Bridges'[21] content-related domain, specifically the impact of proactive palliative consultation on the number of days in the medical ICU, hospital, and from ICU admission to discharge. Significant differences were noted in the length of stay in the ICU (8.96 vs 16.28 days) but not for the other 2 outcomes of interest. One study, by Cheung and colleagues,[49] examined outcomes in the clinician-related domain, namely nursing and ICU intensivist satisfaction, although they also collected data on outcomes in other domains, such as ICU length of stay. No significant differences were noted for the study's outcomes; however, the investigators remarked on several difficulties in feasibility of the research design, participant recruitment, and measurement completion. In addition, a study by Curtis and colleagues,[50] mentioned earlier, was placed in the Aslakson and Bridges[21] family-related domain. This study assessed family ratings of death and dying and satisfaction with care after implementation of a multisite, multicomponent intervention and found no significant differences in any of these outcomes.

Table 3
Representative set of prospective studies of ICU palliative care interventions by outcome domain

Authors and Year	Research Aim/Purpose	Design and Sample/Setting	Intervention	Primary Outcomes	Key Findings
System Related[a]					
Mosenthal et al,[52] 2008	Determine the impact of early, structured communication on end-of-life care practice in the trauma ICU	Single-site, prospective, observational, pre-post study of consecutive patients with trauma admitted to the ICU before (n = 286) and after (n = 367) integration of a structured palliative care intervention	Two-part intervention: • Part I: family bereavement support, assessment of prognosis and patient preferences on ICU admission • Part II: interdisciplinary family meeting within 72 h	Goals-of-care discussions DNR orders Withdrawal of life support	83% of patients received part I and 69% received part II Goals-of-care discussions ↑ from 4% to 36% of patient-days No change in mortality, DNR orders, or withdrawal of life support DNR orders and withdrawal of life support were instituted earlier in hospital course ICU length of stay ↓ in decedents

(continued on next page)

Table 3
(continued)

Authors and Year	Research Aim/Purpose	Design and Sample/Setting	Intervention	Primary Outcomes	Key Findings
Penrod et al,[53] 2011	Determine the impact of a time-triggered palliative care quality improvement initiative on care processes for ICU patients	Multisite, prospective, pre-post study of patients admitted to ICUs with stays of ≥5 d from 5 Veterans' Affairs Medical Centers before (n = 176) and after (n = 239) integration of the intervention	Critical care and palliative care providers trained ICU nurse teams to improve care through auditing, performance feedback, improvement tools, education, and monthly team meetings	Before day 1: identification of medical decision maker, patient's AD status, and CPR preference By day 3: patient and family offered social work and spiritual support By day 5: interdisciplinary family meeting	↑ Identification of medical decision makers (40%–52%) ↓ Determination of AD statues (85%–75%) No change in determination of CPR preferences (81% and 87%) ↑ Offers of social work support (22%–60%) ↑ Offers of spiritual support (35%–45%) ↑ Interdisciplinary family meetings (13%–20%)
Lamba et al,[51] 2012	Determine the impact of early communication with physicians and families on end-of-life care practice in the SICU	Single-site, prospective, observational, pre-post study of consecutive patients having liver transplant admitted to the SICU before (n = 79) and after (n = 104) integration of a palliative care intervention	Two-part intervention: • Part I: family bereavement support, assessment of prognosis and patient preferences on ICU admission • Part II: interdisciplinary family meeting within 72 h	Goals-of-care discussions DNR orders Withdrawal of life support Family perceptions (QODD)	85% of patients received part I and 58% received part II Goals-of-care discussions ↑ from 2% to 38% of patient-days No change in mortality ↑ DNR status (52%–81%) ↑ Withdrawal of life support (35%–68%) Family perceptions: only 5 pre-QODD and 9 post-QODD questionnaires collected (sample too small for statistical analysis)

Black et al,[40] 2013	Examine the impact of a multifaceted behavioral change intervention to improve compliance with communication and palliative care process measures between families and clinicians	Multisite, prospective, single-arm study in 16 adult ICUs in the Rhode Island ICU Collaborative involving 9348 patients over the 21-mo period of intervention integration	A multidisciplinary steering committee: developed and distributed print and Web-based educational materials; recruited and trained local champions at each institution to implement local practice change; facilitated statewide launch meetings; conducted educational outreach meetings at each institution; held monthly conference calls; and oversaw a secure database for data collection and support of routine audit and feedback at an institutional and statewide level	By day 1: medical record documentation of a surrogate decision maker; code status; ADs; completion of a pain assessment; completion of a dyspnea assessment; provision of an ICU brochure By day 3: medical record documentation of a multidisciplinary team meeting; a prognosis discussion; patient-specific goals; completion of an assessment of the need for spiritual care	Day 1 process measure compliance ↑ from 10.7% to 83.8% Day 3 process measure compliance ↑ from 1.6% to 28.8%

(continued on next page)

Table 3
(continued)

Authors and Year	Research Aim/Purpose	Design and Sample/Setting	Intervention	Primary Outcomes	Key Findings
Content Related[b]					
Norton et al,[54] 2007	Examine the effect of proactive palliative care consultation on length of stay for high-risk patients in the medical ICU	Single-site, prospective, pre-post study of seriously ill patients at high risk of dying in a 17-bed medical ICU before (n = 65) and after (n = 126) proactive palliative care consultation	Basic or complete palliative care consultation (see text for details)	Days in the medical ICU Days in the hospital Days from medical ICU admission to discharge	Proactive palliative care patients had significantly shorter medical ICU lengths of stay (8.96 vs 16.28 d) No significant differences in hospital days or days from medical ICU admission to discharge
Clinician Related[c]					
Cheung et al,[49] 2010	Determine whether palliative care teams can improve patient, family, and staff satisfaction for patients receiving end-of-life care in the ICU and reduce surrogate markers of health care costs	Single-site, unblinded, prospective, randomized controlled feasibility trial of terminal and preterminal patients receiving either usual ICU care (n = 10) or usual care plus a palliative care consultation (n = 10)	Palliative care consultation (see text for details)	Nursing staff satisfaction ICU intensivist satisfaction Family satisfaction ICU length of stay Hospital length of stay	No significant differences in all outcomes

Family Related[d]

Curtis et al,[50] 2011	Evaluate the effectiveness of a multidisciplinary quality improvement intervention to improve ICU end-of-life care	Multisite, prospective, unblinded, cluster randomized trial of 12 hospitals (n = 6 intervention, n = 6 control) that included 2318 patients	Five components: 1. Clinician education about ICU palliative care 2. Training of ICU palliative care clinician champions 3. Addressing of barriers to quality end-of-life care by ICU directors 4. Feedback of individual ICU-specific quality data including family satisfaction 5. Implementation of system supports such as palliative care order forms	Family ratings of QODD Family satisfaction with care Nurse-assessed QODD	No change in family QODD scores No change in family satisfaction No change in nurse QODD scores

Abbreviations: AD, advance directive; CPR, cardiopulmonary resuscitation; DNR, do not resuscitate.

[a] For example, percentage of patients with DNR orders, percentage of patients receiving a palliative care consult.

[b] For example, ICU length of stay, time family members speak during a meeting, use of percutaneous gastronomy tubes.

[c] For example, nurse QODD score, health care provider satisfaction score.

[d] For example, hospital anxiety and depression score, ICU family satisfaction, family member of death and dying score.

Data from Refs.[40,49–54]

Several additional points are worth mentioning about the prospective studies in **Table 3**. First, only 2 of these prospective studies specifically examined the direct impact of specialist palliative care clinicians on ICU outcomes.[49,54] Second, there is a dearth of prospective studies in Aslakson and Bridges'[21] content-related, clinician-related, and family-related ICU domains. Third, prospective studies of ICU palliative care have yet to show a measured impact on patient-reported, family-reported, and clinician-reported outcomes. Showing beneficial outcomes through rigorous trials is key to palliative care acceptance and, ultimately, use in the ICU. For example, one survey of clinicians in a trauma ICU reported that they perceived that miscommunication promulgated by palliative care teams was a major barrier to further use of palliative care services; the accuracy of clinician communication during encounters remains an unstudied outcome.[55] Fourth, few if any ICU palliative care prospective trials have specifically targeted patient symptoms (eg, pain, dyspnea, delirium). In addition, intervention details in these studies are sparse, making it difficult assess, adapt, replicate, or translate for clinical application if appropriate.

SUMMARY

ICU patient populations and care complexity span a broad array of diagnoses and acuity levels. Quality-of-care concerns have arisen, especially for patients who are not likely to survive their acute events. Although much of the evaluation of palliative care relies on subjective patient report, families are often the target of care quality improvement because patients may not be conscious toward the end of life. Palliative care has been recommended as a strategy to overcome the quality-of-care issues, and there is early evidence that some aspects of care have been affected when these services have been integrated. However, there is a lack of consensus regarding the outcomes that are of greatest value to measure and how to rigorously do so. A few prospective trials have examined a limited number of outcomes; however, there is disagreement between what is important to patients and families and what clinicians and health systems consider the best targets of palliative care. Overcoming challenges to measuring palliative care outcomes will require consensus development and rigorous research on the best way to evaluate the growing number of programs offering ICU palliative care services.

REFERENCES

1. A controlled trial to improve care for seriously ill hospitalized patients. The Study to Understand Prognoses and Preferences for Outcomes and Risks of Treatments (SUPPORT). The SUPPORT Principal Investigators. JAMA 1995;274(20):1591–8.
2. Field MJ, Cassel CK. Approaching death: improving care at the end of life. Washington, DC: National Academy Press; 1997.
3. Institute of Medicine. Dying in America: Improving quality and honoring individual preferences near the end of life. Washington, DC: The National Academies Press; 2014.
4. Espinosa L, Young A, Symes L, et al. ICU nurses' experiences in providing terminal care. Crit Care Nurs Q 2010;33(3):273–81.
5. Whitehead PB, Herbertson RK, Hamric AB, et al. Moral distress among healthcare professionals: report of an institution-wide survey. J Nurs Scholarsh 2015; 47(2):117–25.
6. Nelson JE, Mathews KS, Weissman DE, et al. Integration of palliative care in the context of rapid response: a report from the improving palliative care in the ICU advisory board. Chest 2015;147(2):560–9.

7. Aslakson RA, Curtis JR, Nelson JE. The changing role of palliative care in the ICU. Crit Care Med 2014;42(11):2418–28.
8. Zalenski R, Courage C, Edelen A, et al. Evaluation of screening criteria for palliative care consultation in the MICU: a multihospital analysis. BMJ Support Palliat Care 2014;4(3):254–62.
9. Arnold RM, Back AL, Barnato AE, et al. The critical care communication project: improving fellows' communication skills. J Crit Care 2015;30(2):250–4.
10. Hua M, Wunsch H. Integrating palliative care in the ICU. Curr Opin Crit Care 2014;20(6):673–80.
11. Bradley CT, Brasel KJ. Developing guidelines that identify patients who would benefit from palliative care services in the surgical intensive care unit. Crit Care Med 2009;37(3):946–50.
12. Hua MS, Li G, Blinderman CD, et al. Estimates of the need for palliative care consultation across United States intensive care units using a trigger-based model. Am J Respir Crit Care Med 2014;189(4):428–36.
13. Aslakson R, Cheng J, Vollenweider D, et al. Evidence-based palliative care in the intensive care unit: a systematic review of interventions. J Palliat Med 2014;17(2): 219–35.
14. Wang L, Piet L, Kenworthy CM, et al. Association between palliative case management and utilization of inpatient, intensive care unit, emergency department, and hospice in Medicaid beneficiaries. Am J Hosp Palliat Care 2015;32(2): 216–20.
15. Khandelwal N, Kross EK, Engelberg RA, et al. Estimating the effect of palliative care interventions and advance care planning on ICU utilization: a systematic review. Crit Care Med 2015;43(5):1102–11.
16. Jang RW, Krzyzanowska MK, Zimmermann C, et al. Palliative care and the aggressiveness of end-of-life care in patients with advanced pancreatic cancer. J Natl Cancer Inst 2015;107(3):dju424.
17. Lautrette A, Ciroldi M, Ksibi H, et al. End-of-life family conferences: rooted in the evidence. Crit Care Med 2006;34(11 Suppl):S364–72.
18. Sadler E, Hales B, Henry B, et al. Factors affecting family satisfaction with inpatient end-of-life care. PLoS One 2014;9(11):e110860.
19. Nelson JE, Bassett R, Boss RD, et al. Models for structuring a clinical initiative to enhance palliative care in the intensive care unit: a report from the IPAL-ICU Project (Improving Palliative Care in the ICU). Crit Care Med 2010;38(9): 1765–72.
20. Penrod JD, Pronovost PJ, Livote EE, et al. Meeting standards of high-quality intensive care unit palliative care: clinical performance and predictors. Crit Care Med 2012;40(4):1105–12.
21. Aslakson RA, Bridges JF. Assessing the impact of palliative care in the intensive care unit through the lens of patient-centered outcomes research. Curr Opin Crit Care 2013;19(5):504–10.
22. Kross EK, Engelberg RA, Downey L, et al. Differences in end-of-life care in the ICU across patients cared for by medicine, surgery, neurology, and neurosurgery physicians. Chest 2014;145(2):313–21.
23. Teno JM, Gozalo PL, Bynum JP, et al. Change in end-of-life care for Medicare beneficiaries: site of death, place of care, and health care transitions in 2000, 2005, and 2009. JAMA 2013;309(5):470–7.
24. Goodman DC, Fisher ES, Chang G-H, et al. Quality of end-of-life cancer care for Medicare beneficiaries: regional and hospital-specific analyses. Lebanon (NH): The Dartmouth Institute for Health Policy and Clinical Practice; 2010.

25. Goodman D, Esty AR, Fisher ES, et al. Trends and variation in end-of-life care for Medicare beneficiaries with severe chronic illness. Lebanon (NH): The Dartmouth Atlas Project; 2011.

26. Morden NE, Chang CH, Jacobson JO, et al. End-of-life care for Medicare beneficiaries with cancer is highly intensive overall and varies widely. Health Aff (Millwood) 2012;31(4):786–96.

27. Menon PR, Stapleton RD, McVeigh U, et al. Telemedicine as a tool to provide family conferences and palliative care consultations in critically ill patients at rural health care institutions: a pilot study. Am J Hosp Palliat Care 2015;32(4):448–53.

28. Kirsh S, Wu WC, Edelman D, et al. Research versus quality improvement: distinct or a distinction without a difference? A case study comparison of two studies. Jt Comm J Qual Patient Saf 2014;40(8):365–75.

29. Rivers E, Nguyen B, Havstad S, et al. Early goal-directed therapy in the treatment of severe sepsis and septic shock. N Engl J Med 2001;345(19):1368–77.

30. Pro CI, Yealy DM, Kellum JA, et al. A randomized trial of protocol-based care for early septic shock. N Engl J Med 2014;370(18):1683–93.

31. National Consensus Project. Clinical practice guidelines for quality palliative care. 3rd edition. Brooklyn (NY): National Consensus Project for Quality Palliative Care; 2013.

32. Enguidanos S, Vesper E, Lorenz K. 30-day readmissions among seriously ill older adults. J Palliat Med 2012;15(12):1356–61.

33. Brumley R, Enguidanos S, Jamison P, et al. Increased satisfaction with care and lower costs: results of a randomized trial of in-home palliative care. J Am Geriatr Soc 2007;55(7):993–1000.

34. Penrod JD, Deb P, Luhrs C, et al. Cost and utilization outcomes of patients receiving hospital-based palliative care consultation. J Palliat Med 2006;9(4):855–60.

35. Bakitas M, Lyons KD, Hegel MT, et al. Effects of a palliative care intervention on clinical outcomes in patients with advanced cancer: the Project ENABLE II randomized controlled trial. JAMA 2009;302(7):741–9.

36. Bakitas M, Tosteson TD, Li Z, et al. Early versus delayed initiation of concurrent palliative oncology care: patient outcomes in the ENABLE III randomized controlled trial. J Clin Oncol 2015;33(13):1438–45.

37. Temel JS, Greer JA, Muzikansky A, et al. Early palliative care for patients with metastatic non-small-cell lung cancer. N Engl J Med 2010;363(8):733–42.

38. Chiarchiaro J, Buddadhumaruk P, Arnold RM, et al. Quality of communication in the ICU and surrogate's understanding of prognosis. Crit Care Med 2015;43(3):542–8.

39. Anderson WG, Cimino JW, Ernecoff NC, et al. A multicenter study of key stakeholders' perspectives on communicating with surrogates about prognosis in intensive care units. Ann Am Thorac Soc 2015;12(2):142–52.

40. Black MD, Vigorito MC, Curtis JR, et al. A multifaceted intervention to improve compliance with process measures for ICU clinician communication with ICU patients and families. Crit Care Med 2013;41(10):2275–83.

41. Curtis JR, Ciechanowski PS, Downey L, et al. Development and evaluation of an interprofessional communication intervention to improve family outcomes in the ICU. Contemp Clin Trials 2012;33(6):1245–54.

42. Quill TE, Abernethy AP. Generalist plus specialist palliative care — creating a more sustainable model. N Engl J Med 2013;368(13):1173–5.

43. Visser M, Deliens L, Houttekier D. Physician-related barriers to communication and patient and family-centred decision making towards the end of life in intensive care: a systematic review. Crit Care 2014;18(6):604.

44. Chen E, McCann JJ, Lateef OB. Attitudes toward and experiences in end-of-life care education in the intensive care unit: a survey of resident physicians. Am J Hosp Palliat Care 2014. [Epub ahead of print].
45. DeCato TW, Engelberg RA, Downey L, et al. Hospital variation and temporal trends in palliative and end-of-life care in the ICU. Crit Care Med 2013;41(6): 1405–11.
46. Lupu D, American Academy of Hospice and Palliative Medicine Workforce Task Force. Estimate of current hospice and palliative medicine physician workforce shortage. J Pain Symptom Manage 2010;40(6):899–911.
47. Donabedian A. 1st edition. An introduction to quality assurance in health care, vol. 1. New York: Oxford University Press; 2003.
48. Agency for Healthcare Research and Quality. AHRQ National Guideline Clearinghouse. 2013. Available at: www.guideline.gov. Accessed December 2, 2013.
49. Cheung W, Aggarwal G, Fugaccia E, et al. Palliative care teams in the intensive care unit: a randomised, controlled, feasibility study. Crit Care Resusc 2010; 12(1):28–35.
50. Curtis JR, Nielsen EL, Treece PD, et al. Effect of a quality-improvement intervention on end-of-life care in the intensive care unit: a randomized trial. Am J Respir Crit Care Med 2011;183(3):348–55.
51. Lamba S, Murphy P, McVicker S, et al. Changing end-of-life care practice for liver transplant service patients: structured palliative care intervention in the surgical intensive care unit. J Pain Symptom Manage 2012;44(4):508–19.
52. Mosenthal AC, Murphy PA, Barker LK, et al. Changing the culture around end-of-life care in the trauma intensive care unit. J Trauma 2008;64(6):1587–93.
53. Penrod JD, Luhrs CA, Livote EE, et al. Implementation and evaluation of a network-based pilot program to improve palliative care in the intensive care unit. J Pain Symptom Manage 2011;42(5):668–71.
54. Norton SA, Hogan LA, Holloway RG, et al. Proactive palliative care in the medical intensive care unit: effects on length of stay for selected high-risk patients. Crit Care Med 2007;35(6):1530–5.
55. Karlekar M, Collier B, Parish A, et al. Utilization and determinants of palliative care in the trauma intensive care unit: results of a national survey. Palliat Med 2014; 28(8):1062–8.

Moving?

Make sure your subscription moves with you!

To notify us of your new address, find your **Clinics Account Number** (located on your mailing label above your name), and contact customer service at:

Email: journalscustomerservice-usa@elsevier.com

800-654-2452 (subscribers in the U.S. & Canada)
314-447-8871 (subscribers outside of the U.S. & Canada)

Fax number: 314-447-8029

Elsevier Health Sciences Division
Subscription Customer Service
3251 Riverport Lane
Maryland Heights, MO 63043

*To ensure uninterrupted delivery of your subscription, please notify us at least 4 weeks in advance of move.

Printed and bound by CPI Group (UK) Ltd, Croydon, CR0 4YY

03/10/2024

01040495-0010